For my husband, Robin Peavler, M.D.

LUCKY ME.

CONTENTS

THE BUSY COUPLE'S GUIDE TO GREAT SEX:

The Medically Proven Program to Boost Low Libido

BY

RALLIE MCALLISTER, MD, MPH, MSEH

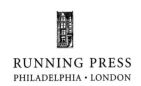

RUNNING PRESS
PHILADELPHIA · LONDON

9 8 7 6 5 4 3 2 1

Digit on the right indicates the number of this printing

Library of Congress Control Number 2003108321

ISBN 0-7624-1832-X

Cover designed by Bill Jones
Interior designed by Jan Greenberg
Edited by Deborah Grandinetti
Typography: Minion and Univers Condensed

This book may be ordered by mail from the publisher.
Please include $2.50.for postage and handling.
But try your bookstore first!

Running Press Book Publishers
125 South Twenty-second Street
Philadelphia, Pennsylvania 19103-4399

Visit us on the web!
www.runningpress.com

ACKNOWLEDGEMENTS

I extend my heartfelt thanks to the following people: Deborah Grandinetti, my editor, for her insight, inspiration, and hard work, and Michael Ward, for making it all possible. To Gayle Santich and Nancy Rectenwald, my sisters and best friends, for their cheerful support, and to Mary Austin, my agent, for always believing in me. My sincere appreciation goes to my colleagues, Cheri Moran, Amy Toney, Jackie Smith, and Keri Austin, for holding down the fort. Special thanks to Deborah Trautman, Pickens Gantt, M.D., Diana Harshbarger, Pharm. D., and Billy Burford, LMT, for their time and expertise, and to all the wonderful people who generously shared the stories of their lives.

■ PART I

CHAPTER 1

TROUBLE
IN PARADISE

NEWS FLASH: THERE'S TROUBLE IN PARADISE.

America, arguably one of the sexiest nations in the entire world, is suffering a serious lag in libido. A report published in the most credible of sources, the *Journal of the American Medical Association* (JAMA), recently unveiled the bad news, baring the sorry state of sexuality in America for all to see.

The *JAMA* sextistics are grim: At first glance, some 43 percent of American women and 31 percent of American men appear to be stricken with some type of sexual inadequacy. Incredibly, diminished desire reportedly affects an estimated 33 percent of women and 17 percent of men. But even in the face of these unthinkable figures, experts speculate that the numbers reflect only the visible tip of a rapidly emerging iceberg. Since cultural taboos and personal embarrassment undoubtedly hinder the ease and accuracy with which people report their perceived sexual shortcomings, these numbers are likely on the low side.

As the news of America's lackluster libido trickled into to the global consciousness, our international neighbors momentarily pondered this curious phenomenon. Back on home turf, however, a number of us did not. In the same breath that carried a heartfelt sigh of relief, many of us uttered, *"Thank God. I thought it was just me."*

With the public tarnishing of America's reputation, other nations boldly, and perhaps even smugly, set out to examine their own sexual state of affairs.

Their research revealed the same depressing trend. Operating on the misery-loves-company policy, sexperts in Canada bemoaned their findings: The majority of Canadians would rather sleep than have sex. Among the work-weary Japanese, sex took a backseat not only to sleeping, but incredibly, to shopping and watching television. Even the French weren't romancing enough to live up to their robust reputation.

The *JAMA* revelation did much to ignite the flames of a new type of sexual revolution that is engulfing the globe: a *libido* revolution. Some forty years after the sexual revolution, we are no longer worried about getting all the sex we desire. Now we're desperately wondering how to *desire* the sex that we get.

Sadly, a lag in libido isn't just a personal problem. It invariably causes considerable distress to the involved—or *uninvolved*—partner. Inhibited desire is by far the most common sexual stumbling block in love relationships, striking a sour note of discord in nearly a third of American couples. Incredibly, one in five married couples engage in sexual intercourse fewer than ten times a year. Surveys show that around 30 percent of unmarried couples in long-standing relationships have sex fewer than ten times annually.

With the recognition that low libido is a pervasive and profoundly disturbing problem, it has recently been elevated to the status of an official medical condition, earning itself the elaborate title "Hypoactive Sexual Desire Disorder (HSDD)." As defined by the American Psychiatric Association, HSDD is a "deficiency or absence of sexual fantasies and desire for sexual activity that causes distress to the individual." The definition is intentionally vague, as the esteemed members of the organization collectively acknowledge that there can be—and are—significant differences in the level of sexual interest among healthy, well-adjusted individuals. Regardless of its official definition, people with HSDD often report feeling sexually flat, or in more serious cases, sexually dead.

The debut of HSDD as an official diagnosis created a stir throughout the global medical community. Doctors and therapists love new diagnoses: They help them pigeonhole patients who have perplexing symptoms into manageable categories, and they facilitate treatment plans. With the minting of a shiny new term for this newly recognized disorder of desire, medical specialists of all types are having a heyday attaching it to their patients.

Being diagnosed with HSDD has mixed blessings. On the one hand, having a real diagnosis provides validation and gives you something concrete to focus on overcoming. On the other hand, being the bearer of a diagnosis like hypoactive sexual desire disorder occasionally undermines recovery by enabling some individuals—not you, of course— to consider the medical diagnosis the end of the story, and then do nothing about it. No doubt that can cause unintended consequences in your intimate relationship.

Hypoactive sexual desire disorder can affect men and women at any stage of adulthood, and its causes are multiple and diverse. The source of your problem—or your partner's—may be very different from the root cause for low libido in the next person. Realize that one-size solutions do not fit all.

UNDERSTANDING THE CAUSES OF HSDD

Although the underlying cause frequently points to an unresolved issue within the relationship, this is not always the case. There can be a multitude of causes—including those that are medical in nature, prescription drug related, or that stem from lifestyle choices. The smartest way to find the most effective solution is to do your own detective work. In the next chapter you will find a series of mini-quizzes designed to help you quickly pinpoint the likely source(s) of the problem.

Common libido zappers include high blood pressure, heart disease, obesity, and hormonal imbalances; the unrecognized side effects of prescription drugs; identity/self-image issues; and sexual trauma. Depression is a major factor, zapping libido in nearly 70 percent of adults diagnosed with the condition. As if that weren't bad enough, many of the modern-day medications commonly used to treat these conditions can leach libido from the lustiest of individuals.

Consider, too, that our lifestyle choices have a dramatic impact on sexuality. Excessive use of tobacco, alcohol, narcotics, and illicit drugs can interfere with libido and sexual performance. The American diet undoubtedly plays a key role as well. Impregnated with fat and loaded with sugar, it makes a hefty contribution to the premature onset of debilitating and deadly diseases. Although diabetes, hardening of the arteries, high blood pressure, and heart disease are the most notorious consequences of our dietary indiscretions, the list includes at least thirty others—many of which can affect sexual functioning, a connection I will make clearer in the chapters ahead.

At the very least, our penchant for rich foods in large quantities leaves us sluggish and sleepy in the short run, and overweight and out of shape in the long run. Dietary overindulgence numbs both the mind and the body to the delicious pleasures of sex, and often douses the desire for it. In the worst cases, it leaves people physically incapable of enjoying it.

While the negative impacts of America's nutritional blasphemy are obvious, other dangers of the American diet are much more insidious. Chemical additives, synthetic preservatives, and trans-fatty acids are detrimental not only to our sexual well-being, but also to our overall health. America's lackluster libido has been attributed to everything from testosterone-lowering artificial sweeteners to estrogen-elevating beef products.

These contributing factors are easy to spot. More insidious, and harder to heal, is the damage caused by internalizing a parent's—or a specific religion's—unhealthy attitudes about sex; or by unhealed pain resulting from prior negative sexual experiences. A competent, professional marriage and family counselor, who has the credentials to serve as a sex therapist, can be of invaluable help in these situations.

Societal Underpinnings of the "Sexless" Society

Social pressures—and certain elements of modern life—also play a role. For many Americans, life in the fast lane is largely responsible for driving away sexual desire. In the aftermath of a crash collision involving several well-defined cultural trends, a prototypical 21st-century couple has emerged. This entity is decidedly businesslike and depressingly sexless.

For starters, the technological revolution, a phenomenon that would supposedly liberate us from work, has ironically enslaved us. Bound to the office by the invisible, invincible ties of cell phones, fax machines, and e-mail, the once-sacred boundaries of the forty-hour workweek no longer exist.

These days, the average American pack mule puts in nearly fifty hours a week, and the already padded workweek is expected to continue to expand over the next decade. As the economy teeters, U.S. businesses are hunkering down, searching for ways to increase efficiency and curb costs. Corporate downsizing is predicted to become even more commonplace in the next decade. Surviving companies will demand more time and greater performance from their employees. Americans will not only work longer, they'll also work harder in an effort to hang on to jobs that are increasingly hard to come by. A recent study revealed that 48 percent of employees feel guilty when they leave work at the end of the day—and not when they leave early, but merely *on time*.

All work and no play can make for a very dull sex life. Job-related stress, which affects an estimated 80 percent of gainfully employed adults, has dire emotional and psychological consequences, as well as biological and physical ones. Stress lowers production of libido-enhancing sex hormones in both men and women, and can ultimately erode sexual performance. Lack of free time leaves less of the precious commodity to spend with partners.

While workaholism creates chronic stress and fatigue in individuals, it also places a tremendous strain on their most important relationships—and their sexuality. Currently, nearly a third of men working more than forty-eight hours a week admit that career pressures significantly hinder their sex lives.

The Extra Burden on Working Parents

Men aren't the only ones working themselves to a frazzle. As much as it pains many women to admit it, the women's liberation movement backfired in several respects. Liberated women are now constitutionally entitled to earn equal pay for equal work. They're free to hold meaningful, high-paying, and high-pressure jobs outside the home. On the flip side, they're also free to work themselves to the point of chronic emotional and physical exhaustion.

While motherhood is still considered a full-time job, it is now perfectly acceptable for the new-generation super-mom to combine it with another, equally demanding career. There are, however, two caveats: First, the super-mom must—at least to some degree—sacrifice her health, happiness, and sense of self. Secondly, she must be aided and abetted by a super-dad who is willing to make a few choice sacrifices of his own.

The high-pressure act of juggling work and family responsibilities eventually takes its toll in the bedroom, where sleep often preempts sex. Working women, especially those with children at home, are subject to mind-boggling stress. Many of them report feeling too fatigued to even think about sex, much less to find the energy to make love.

Nonetheless, the prevalence of working mothers has skyrocketed in the past century. As of 1998, 74 percent of American women had joined the workforce, and the trend of women working outside the home shows no signs of slacking off. It is projected that by 2005, women will comprise nearly half of the nation's total labor force. The hidden cost of all this women's work can be measured in terms of lost intimacy with loved ones; neglect of cherished relationships; and ultimately, the breakdown of the family. Some of this alienation comes as a result of physical separation: Over a third of career women work different shifts than their partners. While absence may indeed create fonder hearts in a few relationships, it more frequently makes finding time to connect as a couple very challenging.

Working couples face another dilemma. Despite the fact that many women put in an equal number of hours on the job as their husbands or partners, there remains a glaring inequality in the division of labor between the sexes. Although modern-day dads are helping out considerably more than their own fathers did, their efforts typically fall far short of their partners'. When it comes to performing child-rearing duties and household chores, women still bear the brunt of the responsibility, and not all of them are happy about it. In fact, there are plenty who harbor resentment over the unequal distribution of labor. These issues can quickly stamp out the flames of desire. Working women who feel under-appreciated and overwhelmed by their myriad roles and responsibilities are less inclined to "reward" their partners with sex.

While stay-at-home moms seem to be less susceptible to the problem of low libido than their working counterparts, they're by no means immune. Many modern-day "housewives" are torn between their maternal obligations and their feelings of self-allegiance. While most of these moms deliberately choose to put their careers on hold while they raise their own children, many experience feelings of anger and jealousy toward their partners. Stay-at-home moms often have difficulty watching their spouses pursue their career goals unfettered, while their own seem to get lost in the wash. Many men who find themselves cast in the role of Mr. Mom experience similar negative emotions. In some cases, these emotions are intensified by an emasculating sense of inadequacy.

The evolution of the American family structure has had a profound negative influence on libido and sexuality. In a society that worships youth above all else, it isn't uncommon to see demanding two-year-olds ruling the roost and calling the shots. Overly-indulged high schoolers typically have hotter cars, nicer threads, and more spending money than their parents had as young working adults. To satisfy these pint-sized and pimply faced consumers, the self-appointed martyrs who produced them are willingly working themselves into the ground, trading huge chunks of their souls—and sexuality—for the almighty paycheck.

While raising children was once treated as a single aspect of a fulfilling marriage, it is now seemingly the sole purpose of the blessed union. Husbands and wives are no longer primarily lovers and companions; they're the harassed and harangued co-directors in the extravagant production of

raising their voracious offspring. These days, parents can expect to spend the majority of their free time carting the fruit of their loins to and from the various places that entitled children must be and be seen: dance classes, music lessons, soccer practice, and dermatology appointments. Children often grow up viewing parents as means to their own ends, and this notion isn't easily dispelled during adolescence, or even adulthood.

Unable to maintain the lavish lifestyle afforded them by their hardworking parents, adult children are leaving the nest later, and in some cases, not at all. These days, many married couples continue to labor long past retirement age to support their fully grown, emotionally stunted adult children.

The Accumulation of the Years

Even without the burden of carrying this extra weight, the ever-increasing life span is taking its toll on the adult sex life. As couples grow older, their bodies—and their relationships—begin to show signs of wear and tear. Sexual desires and drives naturally fade with exposure. More damaging are the unresolved issues between partners that tend to fester over time. The slow, poisonous ooze of anger and resentment can ultimately spell death for intimacy. Even among couples who rate their marriages as happy, the frequency of lovemaking and sexual intercourse naturally tends to decline with age.

More often than not, advancing age is accompanied by a host of medical problems and bewildering physical transformations. Added to the emotional and hormonal changes that go hand in hand with aging, the sexual appetites of even the lustiest individuals are gradually worn away. In a society that unabashedly worships youth and beauty, growing old can be a traumatic, ego-slapping experience. Television shows, magazines, and movies are dominated by malnourished adolescents who fleetingly meet the rigid cultural criteria that define beauty and sex appeal. This barrage of "beauty pornography" from the media and entertainment industries can sabotage the sexual confidence and self-esteem of anyone, but especially of mature adults, no matter how vibrant, healthy, or attractive they might be.

Feeling hopelessly unattractive, emotionally overwhelmed, chronically fatigued, and perpetually stressed out, many once-passionate couples can no longer seem to muster up the motivation, momentum, or magnetism for even the briefest of sexual interludes, even if they manage to find the time or the privacy. Unhappy with their state of affairs, a growing number of libido-depleted adults are voicing their concerns, in terms that their doctors can no longer ignore.

While it is interesting—and even comforting—to know that there are millions of other adults in the same listing boat, the hard reality is that *you* are the only person who can save the ship. While you will undoubtedly benefit from the help and understanding of your partner, your doctors, counselors, or therapists, it is ultimately up to you to restore your libido.

THE GOOD NEWS

Once you uncover and understand the issues that stand between you and the fulfillment of your sexuality, you can take the necessary steps to recover your libido. The key word is "you." In spite of all the miraculous advances in science and medicine, we have yet to discover a magic pill, potion, or product that will transform us into the sensuous and sexual beings that we are meant to be. If the transformation is to occur in your own mind and body, you must be willing to make the journey, using all the resources you have, including this book. No doubt you'll encounter some roadblocks or detours, but expect the ride to be exciting, energizing, and enlightening. Take my word, it's worth it: The view from the heights is absolutely breathtaking.

If you've been there before, you know how magnificent it is. This exhilarating experience belongs in the panorama of your life. As a sexual, sensuous human being, you were unquestionably designed to receive it—and give it—in full measure.

CHAPTER 2

ZEROING IN ON YOUR "DESIRE" DEFLATORS:

A Self Test for Couples

WHEN MY PATIENT JANICE[1] CAME TO MY OFFICE FOR HER YEARLY CHECKUP, she admitted that she didn't enjoy sex as much as she once had. Because it was less pleasurable, she had begun to avoid making love to her husband.

"It's causing problems in our relationship," she told me. "Charles thinks it's his fault. He keeps asking me what it is that he's done to change my feelings for him. He can't seem to accept the fact that I just don't want to have sex as often as I did a few years ago."

Janice had gone through menopause eight years earlier, at the age of fifty. She had initially taken estrogen replacement therapy to help with the hot flashes, but stopped taking it after about a year. In the past several years, she had begun to experience vaginal dryness, and she agreed that this might be part of the problem.

"It's getting to the point that sex is painful," she said. "After we make love, I stay swollen for days."

With the exception of significant vaginal dryness, Janice's physical examination was normal. Her lab reports were normal as well. As expected, her estrogen and testosterone levels were low, but within the acceptable range for a menopausal woman.

Although oral estrogen replacement therapy would have undoubtedly helped reverse some of Janice's vaginal dryness, she didn't want to take hor-

---

1. All the names of patients have been changed.

mone pills again. Her best friend had died of breast cancer, and she was wary about taking any medicine that might increase her own chances of developing the disease. Janice was, however, willing to try a vaginal cream that contained estrogen. Used just three times a week, the cream helps rejuvenate the cells of the vagina, reversing much of the thinning that occurs with age, and increasing their production of natural secretions. Because the estrogen exerts mainly a localized effect, it's less associated with breast cancer, a fact that made Janice comfortable using it.

When I saw her back at the office for a recheck six months later, Janice told me she was pleased with the results. "I'm not exactly a sex machine," she laughed, "but Charles and I are making love a lot more often than we used to. Now that it doesn't hurt, I really enjoy it."

· · ·

Bill came to see me on a mission: He wanted a prescription for Viagra, and he was determined not to leave without it. When I asked him if he was having trouble achieving an erection, his answer was revealing: "It's not so much the erection that I'm worried about, it's my sex drive. I never thought I'd say this, but I'm really not all that interested in sex anymore."

When I told Bill that Viagra might work to improve his erections, but wouldn't do much to enhance his libido, he was gravely disappointed.

"You mean this is it? It's over?" he asked incredulously.

I reassured him that there might be an explanation for his diminished libido, with a number of possible treatment options. Since Bill was generally healthy and didn't take any medications, I told him that it was entirely possible that his testosterone level was low, and that this might be contributing to his lack of sexual desire. It was the only way I could talk him into having his blood drawn. Loss of libido in men is one of the surest signs of testosterone deficiency, and at sixty-four; Bill was at the right age for andropause.

As suspected, Bill's testosterone level was quite low. After discussing his options for testosterone replacement therapy and reluctantly agreeing to twice yearly blood tests, Bill quickly nixed the testosterone injections and decided to try the patches instead. He got excellent results.

"I feel like I'm twenty years younger," he said. "My sex drive is back, and that's great. But I've also got more energy than I've had in years, and for the first time in a long time, I'm really enjoying life."

• • •

For some young women, ironically enough, birth control pills can be responsible for zapping libido. At twenty-four, Ashley had been taking the Pill for five years. She hadn't noticed any effect on her sex drive until she and her fiancé had been dating for over a year. Ashley had started out taking a monophasic pill, a version that is notorious for dampening sexual desire, so I prescribed a newer triphasic pill, a formulation that is associated with fewer sexual side effects. After three months, Ashley's sex drive was still lacking, and she was getting a little depressed about it.

"I've got to do something," she said, her voice betraying a bit of desperation. "Jordon and I are going to Hawaii on our honeymoon, and he asked me if I thought I'd be in the mood to make love while we were there. He jokes about getting the honeymoon suite with twin beds. He's just kidding around, but I can tell it really bothers him."

Although Ashley's free testosterone level was normal for her age, her libido was not. With this in mind, I offered her the option of using supplemental testosterone to increase her sex drive. After she was convinced that she wouldn't have to shave her chin for her wedding photos, she agreed to try using a testosterone cream, which she could apply to a thin-skinned area of her body several times a week.

Since I wouldn't see Ashley until after her honeymoon, I asked her to give me a call and let me know how her treatment was working. She left a message with my nurse: "Twin beds will not be necessary in Hawaii!"

As a family physician who cares for hundreds of patients a year, I have seen over and over again the heartbreaking consequences of one partner's low sexual desire on his or her intimate relationship. To help my patients prevent the deterioration of this significant relationship, I have learned to ask them, "Are you happy with your sex life?"

Of course, I'm always happy when I receive a positive response. Yet I am *not* surprised when I don't get one. Because sexuality is so complex, and because its expression generally involves two people, there's plenty of opportunity for things to go wrong.

Some of my patients who experience loss of libido come to me on their own, searching for an explanation—and hopefully a solution. Others come reluctantly, often in response to their partners' desperate pleas, a sure sign that diminished desire is straining the relationship. A few of my patients seem determined to suffer in silence, and probably wouldn't discuss the matter if I didn't bring it up. That's unfortunate, because there are often very simple solutions. It's just a matter of determining the problem, then thinking through the best way to remedy it.

Since I am speaking to you from this printed page, rather than sitting down with you in my examining room, let me walk you through the diagnostic process I use with my patients so you'll know the key questions to ask yourself.

Of course, I am *not* advising you to diagnose yourself *instead of* consulting your doctor. What I *am* showing you is how to identify the possible and likely culprits so you can make the most of your next visit with your physician.

When I am examining a patient who tells me that sexual activity isn't as desirable or enjoyable as it once was, I ask specific questions. These are good questions to ask yourself:
- Is it because sexual intercourse is painful?
- Are relationship problems to blame?
- Could it be due to a side effect of a medication?
- Is it caused by fatigue or depression, or by a medical condition?

If the problem isn't easily explained, a complete physical exam and a few blood tests are in order. Women should have breast and pelvic exams, a Pap smear, and a mammogram if their age and history indicate a need for it. Men should have genital and rectal exams. If a patient's sexual complaints seem to point to underlying heart disease, a complete cardiac work-up is necessary. This work-up may include an electrocardiogram (EKG), a cardiac stress test, or an echocardiogram, a study that uses ultrasound technology to determine the function of the heart.

Occasionally, blood tests reveal the reason for the sexual dysfunction, and point to the solution. But even if the blood tests are perfectly normal, they're still necessary. This is because physicians generally do not want to initiate treatment before taking a look at a patient's baseline blood chemistry.

These are the tests I order:
- *Glucose level*: A high fasting glucose level is suggestive of diabetes, although other tests may be necessary to make the diagnosis. Untreated diabetes can cause fatigue, resulting in a diminished sex drive. It is also notorious for causing sexual dysfunction in men and women.

- *Complete blood count*: This test can identify anemia, a blood disorder that can cause fatigue and weakness.
- *Cholesterol level and lipid profile*: High cholesterol levels and an abnormal lipid profile can be indicative of underlying artery disease, which in turn can lead to sexual dysfunction. It's important to measure a patient's baseline lipid status for another reason: Hormone replacement therapies can negatively impact the lipid profile. About six months after starting testosterone replacement therapy, cholesterol level and lipid panel will be rechecked and compared to baseline measurements.
- *Thyroid function test*: Thyroid function influences sex hormone production and regulation. An abnormal thyroid hormone panel is occasionally responsible for low libido or sexual dysfunction.
- *Liver function tests*: Since the liver is involved in regulating sex hormones, it is important to evaluate its state of health. Oral testosterone and DHEA supplements can impact the liver, so it is necessary to obtain baseline measurements for future comparison.
- *Prolactin level*: Occasionally, a tumor in the pituitary gland is responsible for secreting abnormally high levels of prolactin, a hormone that can interfere with the production of estrogen and testosterone. In men and women, high prolactin levels are associated with diminished sexual desire and performance.
- *Follicle stimulating hormone*: This hormone is typically elevated in women who are menopausal or peri-menopausal, and in men who are andropausal or peri-andropausal.
- *Free testosterone level*: This blood test measures the amount of bioavailable testosterone in the body, or the amount of the hormone that is capable of exerting its effects on target glands and tissues. In both men and women, low levels of free testosterone can be at the root of desire and performance problems.
- *Estrogen level*: In women, low estrogen levels typically signal menopause. The test is also useful in men. Occasionally, a man will have a normal testosterone level and an elevated estrogen level, and this combination can interfere with libido and sexual performance.
- *DHEAS level*: DHEAS is manufactured by the adrenal gland in both men and women, and it is the hormone from which estrogen and testosterone are made. If DHEAS levels are low, supplementation with DHEA may be a viable strategy for boosting libido and sexual function.

- *Human growth hormone level (GH)* : In men and women, human growth hormone triggers the production of the sex hormones, specifically testosterone. Especially in older individuals, low levels of GH are often at the root of a waning sex drive. Although GH supplementation is an expensive treatment option, it is usually very effective.
- *Prostate specific antigen (PSA)*: An elevated PSA level may be indicative of prostate cancer, and it is a useful screening test for men over forty. A baseline measurement is also necessary for men who are considering testosterone or GH replacement therapy, since supplemental testosterone and GH may drive up PSA levels in some men.
- *Pregnancy test*: Just in case, for all women of reproductive age.

BARRIERS TO SEXUALITY (BTS) SELF-TEST

Sexuality is very complex. Its full expression is dependent on a number of factors, including physical and emotional health, hormonal balance, diet and exercise habits, and relationship issues. Since a problem in any one of these areas can influence or interfere with your sexuality, it is helpful to evaluate each of them for signs of trouble. The **Barriers To Sexuality (BTS) Self-Test** is designed to help you uncover the problems that may be lowering your libido and preventing you from achieving sexual fulfillment.

I have divided the BTS Self-Test into eight phases. Each phase is designed to assess a different aspect of your sexuality. For the questions included in BTS 1 through 35, simply answer "yes" or "no."

If you would like your partner to take this test as well, you will find a second copy in the appendix.

Barriers To Sexuality (BTS)
Phase I (Men and Women)

■ BTS 1

Yes	No	Are you a man older than forty-five?
Yes	No	Are you a post-menopausal woman?
Yes	No	Do you have a family history of heart disease?
Yes	No	Do you smoke?
Yes	No	Do you have high cholesterol levels?
Yes	No	Do you have high blood pressure?
Yes	No	Are you sedentary?
Yes	No	Are you overweight?
Yes	No	Do you have uncontrolled diabetes?
Yes	No	Do you experience shortness of breath or chest pain with exertion?

■ BTS 2

Yes	No	Does diabetes run in your family?
Yes	No	Are you overweight, especially around the waist?
Yes	No	Do you have excessive thirst or hunger?
Yes	No	Do you urinate frequently?
Yes	No	Do you have blurred vision?
Yes	No	Do you feel extremely fatigued on a regular basis?
Yes	No	Do you have wounds that are slow to heal?
Yes	No	Do you suffer frequent infections of your skin, urinary tract, or vagina?
Yes	No	Do you experience numbness or tingling of your hands or feet?
Yes	No	Does your mouth frequently feel dry?

■ BTS 3

Yes	No	Do you have diabetes?
Yes	No	Do you eat junk food on a regular basis?
Yes	No	Do you eat red meat more than three times a week?
Yes	No	Do you usually eat whole dairy products instead of the low-fat or reduced-fat varieties?
Yes	No	Do you have high blood pressure?
Yes	No	Are you overweight?
Yes	No	Do you rarely exercise?
Yes	No	Do you have trouble achieving or maintaining an erection (men) or becoming or remaining physically aroused (women)?
Yes	No	Have you had your cholesterol levels checked in the past three years?

■ BTS 4

Yes	No	Are you overweight?
Yes	No	Are you older than thirty-five?
Yes	No	Are you of African descent?
Yes	No	Did your mother or sister suffer a heart attack or stroke before the age of fifty-five?
Yes	No	Did your father or brother suffer a heart attack or stroke before the age of forty-five?
Yes	No	Do you exercise less than thirty minutes a day, three to four times a week?
Yes	No	Do you smoke?
Yes	No	Do you eat more than one teaspoon of salt a day?
Yes	No	Do you drink more than two alcoholic beverages per day?
Yes	No	Do you experience frequent, pulsating headaches?

■ BTS 5

Yes	No	Are you gaining weight for no apparent reason?
Yes	No	Are you unable to lose weight with diet and exercise?
Yes	No	Do you suffer from excessive constipation?
Yes	No	Do you feel cold when others do not?
Yes	No	Do you frequently feel fatigued or sluggish?
Yes	No	Is your hair dry, coarse, breaking, or falling out?
Yes	No	Is your skin dry and scaly?
Yes .	No	Do you have puffiness and swelling around your face and eyes?
Yes	No	Do you have difficulty concentrating or remembering things?
Yes	No	Is your sex drive lower than it used to be?

■ BTS 6

Yes	No	Do you feel like your heart is racing or skipping beats?
Yes	No	Do your hands shake?
Yes	No	Do you feel hot, even when others feel cold?
Yes	No	Have you lost weight, even though your appetite is normal or increased?
Yes	No	Do you frequently feel nervous or irritated?
Yes	No	Do you have diarrhea, or loose, frequent bowel movements?
Yes	No	Are you having difficulty getting to sleep, staying asleep, or going back to sleep after awakening in the night?
Yes	No	Do your eyes appear to be larger or more prominent than they used to?
Yes	No	Is your sex drive lower than it once was?
Yes	No	Are you experiencing sexual performance problems?

Yes	No	Are you between the ages of twenty-five to forty-five?
Yes	No	Have you had mononucleosis (mono)?
Yes	No	Have you had severe fatigue that has lasted at least six months and does not seem to improve with rest?
Yes	No	Is your fatigue interfering with your daily activities?
Yes	No	Is your throat frequently sore?
Yes	No	Do you have tender lymph nodes in your neck or under your arms?
Yes	No	Do you have joint pain or muscle pain?
Yes	No	Do you have frequent headaches?
Yes	No	Do you awaken from sleep feeling tired?
Yes	No	Do you have fatigue after light exercise or exertion?

THE ROLE OF HORMONAL IMBALANCE

Sometimes, a loss of sexual desire can be attributed to a hormonal imbalance that involves hormones other than testosterone and estrogen. When Myra complained of loss of libido, she voiced her belief that the problem was largely due to her fatigue. "I'm always so tired. I just don't have the energy to make love—I'd much rather take a nap." Myra's thyroid profile revealed slightly low levels of thyroid hormones, which undoubtedly accounted for her fatigue and contributed to her diminished sexual desire. After she began taking Synthroid, a thyroid hormone replacement medication, her energy levels—and her sex drive—returned to normal.

■ BTS 8

Yes	No	Has your partner told you that you snore when you sleep?
Yes	No	Have you been told that you stop breathing or gasp for air while you're sleeping?
Yes	No	Are you overweight?
Yes	No	Do you have a thick neck or a double chin?

Yes	No	Do you feel tired and sluggish during the day?
Yes	No	Do you feel as if you could easily take a nap during the day?
Yes	No	Do you have trouble staying awake during the day?
Yes	No	Do you fall asleep unexpectedly during the day?
Yes	No	Are you more irritable than you once were?
Yes	No	Has your doctor told you that you have large tonsils, nasal polyps, or a deviated nasal septum?

■ BTS 9

Yes	No	Do you take a prescription or over the counter medication?
Yes	No	Do you feel that you aren't sure about all of the potential side effects of your medication?
Yes	No	Have you noticed that you feel differently since you began taking your medication?
Yes	No	Have you noticed a decrease in sexual desire since you began taking your medication?
Yes	No	Have you noticed a reduction in sexual performance since you began taking your medication?
Yes	No	Do you find that sex is less enjoyable since you began taking your medication?
Yes	No	Do you drink grapefruit juice one or more times per week?

■ BTS 10 (Women)

Yes	No	Are you older than thirty-five?
Yes	No	Do you suffer from frequent urinary tract infections?
Yes	No	Do you have diabetes?
Yes	No	Are you menopausal?
Yes	No	Have you had more than two children?
Yes	No	Do you drink more than three caffeine-containing beverages a day?
Yes	No	Do you experience loss of urine when coughing, sneezing, or laughing?
Yes	No	Do you feel the need to urinate frequently?
Yes	No	Do you experience a sudden, urgent need to urinate?
Yes	No	Have you had abdominal or pelvic surgery?

■ BTS 11 (Men)

Yes	No	Are you older than fifty?
Yes	No	Do you have trouble starting urination?
Yes	No	Do you have a weak flow of urine?
Yes	No	Do you experience dribbling after urination?
Yes	No	Do you feel that your bladder is not completely empty after urinating?
Yes	No	Do you have the urge to go again soon after urinating?
Yes	No	Do you have pain during urination?
Yes	No	Do you wake at night to urinate?
Yes	No	Do you have frequent urination?
Yes	No	Do you experience sudden, uncontrollable urges to urinate?

Barriers to Sexuality
Phase II (Men and Women)

■ BTS 12

Yes	No	Do you feel sad or down most of the day, nearly every day?
Yes	No	Do you have less interest in the activities that you normally enjoy?
Yes	No	Have you lost or gained weight, or noticed a change in appetite?
Yes	No	Are you sleeping too little or too much?
Yes	No	Do you often feel hopeless or worthless?
Yes	No	Do you think about dying or killing yourself?
Yes	No	Do you cry easily?
Yes	No	Do you have trouble remembering things?
Yes	No	Do you have a family history of depression?
Yes	No	Do you have less interest in having sex than you once did?

MAYBE IT'S THE PROZAC . . .

Menopausal women are especially prone to loss of libido, but younger women aren't immune to the problem. At the tender age of thirty-five, Sherry told me that she didn't care if she ever had sex again.

"I'm only here today because my husband made the appointment," she said. "He's getting pretty desperate."

As we discussed the problem, it became clear that Sherry didn't experience pain with intercourse, and she hadn't had any traumatic sexual experiences. She denied having serious relationship problems with her husband. "Except when it comes to sex," she told me. "I just don't think about it. If Paul didn't bring it up, I don't think it would ever occur to me."

A review of her medications revealed that Sherry had been taking Prozac for a little over twelve years. She was pleased when I told her that the medication might be responsible for her diminished desire. She was definitely willing to try going off the Prozac.

"I really don't think I need it anymore," she said. "I started taking it when the kids were young—I got really depressed about being stuck at home with two babies. I think I'll be okay without it now."

Sherry's physical examination and blood tests were all normal, increasing the likelihood that her antidepressant was at the root of the problem. I devised a tapering dosing schedule that would allow her to gradually wean herself off of the medication over a three-week period, and asked her to return to my office in three months for a follow-up appointment.

When I saw her next, Sherry admitted that she might be a little moodier than she had been while she was taking Prozac, but she was able to manage her emotions. She was amazed at the change in her sex drive.

"About two weeks after I took my last pill, I noticed a huge difference. One day I was sitting at work, and I found myself thinking about sex. It just popped into my head. I couldn't remember the last time that had happened. I called my husband and told him that I wanted him really, *really* bad. He had a softball game after work, but he blew it off and came home with a dozen red roses."

Sherry was also delighted to find that she was able to achieve orgasm once she stopped taking her antidepressant.

"I never associated it with the medicine," she told me. "I thought I was one of those women who just couldn't have an orgasm. Now that I know it's always a possibility, I'm much more creative when Paul and I make love!"

■ BTS 13

Yes	No	Do you frequently feel sad, angry, or irritated?
Yes	No	Do you suffer frequent upper respiratory infections?
Yes	No	Do you have trouble falling asleep or staying asleep?
Yes	No	Have you had a recent change in appetite?
Yes	No	Do you have less interest in sex than you once did?
Yes	No	Do you feel that your life is getting out of control?
Yes	No	Are you having trouble concentrating or remembering?

■ BTS 14

Yes	No	When you look at yourself in the mirror, are you dissatisfied with your reflection?
Yes	No	Do you find some aspect of your appearance unacceptable?
Yes	No	Do you wear clothes that hide some part of your body?
Yes	No	Do you sometimes avoid certain social events because of your appearance?
Yes	No	Do you feel that you spend too much time worrying about your weight or appearance?
Yes	No	Do you find that you need frequent reassurance about your weight or appearance?
Yes	No	Are you ashamed of your body or your appearance?
Yes	No	Do you wish that you could have cosmetic surgery to correct some flaw in your appearance?
Yes	No	Did your family or friends criticize your weight or appearance when you were a child?

Barriers to Sexuality Phase III

■ BTS 15 (Women)

Around the time of your menstrual period:

Yes	No	Do you experience bloating or weight gain?
Yes	No	Are your breasts tender?
Yes	No	Do you feel anxious or irritable?
Yes	No	Do you cry more easily than usual?

Yes	No	Do you feel excessively tired?
Yes	No	Do you experience food cravings or changes in your appetite?
Yes	No	Do you sleep more or less than you usually do?
Yes	No	Do you have trouble concentrating or remembering things?
Yes	No	Do you experience abdominal pain or changes in your bowel habits?
Yes	No	Do you find that you're less interested in sex than usual?

■ BTS 16 (Women)

Yes	No	Do you have hot flashes?
Yes	No	Do you have breast tenderness?
Yes	No	Have your PMS symptoms worsened?
Yes	No	Do you have decreased libido?
Yes	No	Are your periods irregular?
Yes	No	Do you suffer from fatigue?
Yes	No	Do you have vaginal dryness or discomfort during sex?
Yes	No	Do you have urine leakage when coughing or sneezing?
Yes	No	Do you have mood swings?
Yes	No	Are you having difficulty sleeping?

■ BTS 17 (Women)

Have you ceased menstruating?

Yes	No	Are you suffering from hot flashes?
Yes	No	Do you have mood swings?
Yes	No	Do you have less interest in sex than you used to?
Yes	No	Are you having trouble sleeping?
Yes	No	Do you have a rapid or irregular heartbeat at times?
Yes	No	Are you having joint pain or headaches?
Yes	No	Are you having trouble remembering or concentrating?
Yes	No	Do you experience vaginal dryness and itching, or an increased number of vaginal infections?
Yes	No	Do you experience pain during intercourse?

THE TESTOSTERONE LINK IN WOMEN

Libby was menopausal, but vaginal dryness wasn't responsible for her lack of libido. She had been taking estrogen replacement therapy for two years, and she wasn't bothered by the classic menopausal symptoms.

"The only real change I've noticed is in my sex drive," she said. "I love being with my husband. I like to cuddle and hold hands, but I have absolutely no desire to make love to him."

Libby's hormone profile revealed the expected. The supplemental estrogen had boosted her estrogen level, but her free testosterone level was quite low. Although this is a "normal" finding in menopausal women, it is often responsible for diminished sexual desire.

Libby was anxious to try just about anything to increase her sex drive. We discussed using a testosterone cream to boost her testosterone level, but since she was already taking an estrogen pill, she opted to switch to Estratest, a pill that contains a balanced mix of both estrogen and testosterone. For Libby, the combination was very effective in restoring her sexual desire.

■ BTS 18 (Women)

Yes	No	Are you older than forty-five?
Yes	No	Are you menopausal?
Yes	No	Have you been diagnosed with osteoporosis?
Yes	No	Have you noticed that you're less interested in sex than you once were?
Yes	No	Have you noticed that you rarely think or fantasize about sex?
Yes	No	Do you enjoy sex less than you once did?
Yes	No	Do you have trouble remembering or concentrating more than you once did?
Yes	No	Are you less muscular than you once were?
Yes	No	Do you feel as if your muscles are weaker than they once were?
Yes	No	Have you noticed an increase in your body fat?

Yes	No	Do you frequently experience fatigue for no apparent reason?
Yes	No	Have your moods been depressed lately?
Yes	No	Have you been more irritable recently?
Yes	No	Are you less focused than you once were?
Yes	No	Do you look less muscular than you once did?
Yes	No	Do you feel as if you're not as strong as you once were?
Yes	No	Do you have more body fat than you once did?
Yes	No	Is your sex drive lower than it once was?
Yes	No	Are you having difficulty achieving or maintaining an erection?
Yes	No	Do you have less facial and body hair than you once did?

Barriers to Sexuality
Phase IV (Men and Women)

■ BTS 20

Yes	No	Do you drink alcoholic beverages on a regular basis?
Yes	No	Do you ever find yourself wishing that you could cut down or drink less?
Yes	No	Do you ever find yourself getting angry when someone suggests that you drink less?
Yes	No	Do you ever feel guilty about your drinking?
Yes	No	Do you ever take a drink in the morning as an "eye-opener" or to help you recover from a hangover?

■ BTS 21

Yes	No	Do you find that you're out of breath after climbing a flight of stairs?
Yes	No	Are you frequently tired, even when you haven't engaged in strenuous activity?
Yes	No	Do you find it difficult or impossible to touch your toes?
Yes	No	Do you seldom or rarely exercise?
Yes	No	Do you usually take the elevator instead of the stairs?

Yes	No	Do you feel that you're less energetic than you used to be?
Yes	No	Are you overweight?
Yes	No	Do you feel that you're weaker than you used to be?

■ BTS 22

Yes	No	Do you routinely sleep less than seven hours a night?
Yes	No	Do you feel as if you could easily fall asleep at almost any time during the day?
Yes	No	Do you find yourself nodding off unexpectedly?
Yes	No	Do you feel that you're more irritable lately?
Yes	No	Do you frequently feel tired and run-down during the day?
Yes	No	Do you feel exhausted and ready for bed long before your partner is?
Yes	No	Do you have trouble concentrating?
Yes	No	Are you more forgetful than you once were?
Yes	No	Do you find it difficult to get out of bed in the morning?
Yes	No	Do you feel that you're usually too tired to have sex?

■ BTS 23

Yes	No	Do you routinely work more than ten hours a day?
Yes	No	Do you find yourself thinking about work when you should be relaxing?
Yes	No	Do you spend your free time on work-related projects?
Yes	No	Do you carry a work-related cell phone or a pager, even when you're "off-duty?"
Yes	No	Has your work ever caused you to miss an important social or family obligation?
Yes	No	Has your work ever caused you to break a promise?
Yes	No	Has your partner ever complained that your job comes before him/her?

■ BTS 24

Yes	No	Do you regularly skip breakfast?
Yes	No	Do you rarely eat three meals a day?
Yes	No	Do you usually eat more than three snacks a day?
Yes	No	Do you frequently skip meals?
Yes	No	Do you find that you are often so hungry that you overeat at mealtime?
Yes	No	Do you eat most of your meals somewhere besides a dining table?
Yes	No	Do you eat more than three meals a week at fast food restaurants?
Yes	No	Do you frequently eat on the go?
Yes	No	Do you frequently graze, or eat continuously?

■ BTS 25

Yes	No	Do you eat fewer than three servings of fruit each day?
Yes	No	Do you eat fewer than three servings of vegetables each day?
Yes	No	Are you on a high-protein diet?
Yes	No	Do you frequently experience food cravings?
Yes	No	Do you often feel sluggish or sleepy after you eat?
Yes	No	Do you often feel hungry soon after eating?
Yes	No	Do you drink fewer than six glasses of water a day?

■ BTS 26

Yes	No	Do you drink more than three cups of regular coffee a day?
Yes	No	Do you drink more than three caffeine-containing soft drinks a day?
Yes	No	Do you find that you're nervous or irritable if you miss your morning coffee?
Yes	No	Do you develop a headache when you miss your morning coffee?
Yes	No	Do you usually drink a cup of coffee or a caffeine-containing soft drink for a "pick me up" during the day?
Yes	No	Do you awaken with a headache on the mornings that you sleep in?

Barriers To Sexuality
Phase V (Men and Women)

■ BTS 27

Yes	No	Do you have less interest in sex than you once did?
Yes	No	Do you find that you rarely or never think or fantasize about sex?
Yes	No	Do you find that you rarely or never initiate sex with your partner?
Yes	No	Do you have sex just to please your partner?
Yes	No	Has your partner expressed concern about your lack of sexual desire?
Yes	No	Is your lack of sexual desire causing problems in your relationship?
Yes	No	Do you wish that you were more interested in sex?
Yes	No	Have you ever experienced a traumatic sexual encounter?
Yes	No	Were you taught as a child that sex is shameful or sinful?

■ BTS 28

Yes	No	Do you have little interest in sex?
Yes	No	Do you rarely or never experience orgasm with sexual intercourse?
Yes	No	Are you rarely or never able to achieve orgasm by any means?
Yes	No	Do you take an antidepressant or sedative medication?
Yes	No	Do you have a history of drug or alcohol abuse?

■ BTS 29 (Women)

Yes	No	Do you suffer from depression or anxiety?
Yes	No	Do you have a chronic illness, like heart disease, lung disease, or diabetes?
Yes	No	Do you have a history of drug or alcohol abuse?
Yes	No	Do you take antidepressant medications?
Yes	No	Are you having marital or relationship problems?

Yes	No	Do you have a history of sexual abuse?
Yes	No	Are you unable to experience orgasm?
Yes	No	Do you experience pain during sexual intercourse?
Yes	No	Do you have little interest in having sex?
Yes	No	Do you feel that you have inadequate vaginal lubrication?

■ BTS 30 (Women)

Yes	No	Do you have pelvic pain with intercourse, especially when your partner thrusts?
Yes	No	Are you menopausal?
Yes	No	Do you suffer from frequent vaginal infections?
Yes	No	Have you had a C-section?
Yes	No	Have you had a hysterectomy?
Yes	No	Have you had a bilateral tubal ligation (tubes tied)?
Yes	No	Have you had abdominal surgery?
Yes	No	Have you ever been diagnosed with pelvic inflammatory disease?
Yes	No	Has it been more than two years since you had a pelvic exam?
Yes	No	Do you suffer from vaginal dryness?

■ BTS 31 (Women)

Yes	No	Do you experience vaginal pain with penetration?Do you feel that penetration is difficult or impossible at times?
Yes	No	Do you fear that sexual intercourse will be painful?
Yes	No	Do you have a history of sexual trauma, including rape or sexual abuse as a child?
Yes	No	Have you ever experienced feelings of panic or extreme anxiety prior to or during sexual intercourse?

■ BTS 32 (Men)

Yes	No	Are you younger than thirty?
Yes	No	Do you frequently ejaculate before you want to?
Yes	No	Do you usually experience orgasm before your partner does?
Yes	No	Do you feel that you are unable to stop yourself from climaxing, even for a few seconds?
Yes	No	Were you taught as a child that sex is shameful or sinful?
Yes	No	Do you frequently experience feelings of guilt about having sex?

■ BTS 33 (Men)

Yes	No	Do you sometimes fail to get an erection during sexual activity?
Yes	No	Do you sometimes fail to maintain an erection during sexual activity?
Yes	No	Do you feel that your erection is less firm than it once was?
Yes	No	Do you feel that you are having problems or turmoil in your relationship?
Yes	No	Do you smoke?
Yes	No	Are you older than fifty?
Yes	No	Do you have diabetes?
Yes	No	Do you have high blood pressure?
Yes	No	Do you have high cholesterol?
Yes	No	Do you take medication for depression, high cholesterol, or high blood pressure?

Barriers to Sexuality Phase VI

■ BTS 34 (Men)

Yes	No	I have a hard time making small talk with my partner.
Yes	No	When my partner tells me about her problems, I find myself offering her solutions instead of encouraging her to discuss them.
Yes	No	I tend to "show" my partner my love, rather than "tell" her.
Yes	No	I have trouble discussing my feelings with my partner.
Yes	No	I feel that making love is a reasonable substitute for conversation.

■ BTS 35 (Women)

Yes	No	I try to engage my partner in small talk, even when he's not in the mood for conversation.
Yes	No	I try to get my partner to "open up" and discuss his problems or concerns, even if it makes him uncomfortable.
Yes	No	I tend to tell my partner that I love him more often than I show him.
Yes	No	I think conversation is a reasonable substitute for making love.

Barriers to Sexuality
Phase VII (Men and Women)

To answer the questions for BTS 36 through BTS 45, circle the number that reflects the following statements:

1—Strongly agree
2—Somewhat agree
3—Neither agree nor disagree
4—Somewhat disagree
5—Strongly disagree

■ BTS 36

1	2	3	4	5	My usual sexual encounter is a "quickie."
1	2	3	4	5	I find it difficult to make time in my schedule to make love to my partner.
1	2	3	4	5	Sex is last on my "to do" list.
1	2	3	4	5	I rarely think about making love to my partner.
1	2	3	4	5	I hardly ever initiate sexual activity.

■ BTS 37

1	2	3	4	5	I do not think of myself as being a sexual person.
1	2	3	4	5	I seldom wear clothes that make me feel sexy.
1	2	3	4	5	I do not flirt with my partner.
1	2	3	4	5	I rarely have sexual thoughts or fantasies.
1	2	3	4	5	I'm not sure what it takes to make me feel sexy.

■ BTS 38

1	2	3	4	5	Having sex feels like a chore.
1	2	3	4	5	When my partner and I make love, I know just what to expect.
1	2	3	4	5	My partner and I make love in the same location.
1	2	3	4	5	My partner and I rarely try new sexual positions.
1	2	3	4	5	I find it difficult to get excited about having sex with my partner.

■ BTS 39

1	2	3	4	5	My partner and I rarely spend time alone with each other.
1	2	3	4	5	When my partner and I are together, we usually talk about our jobs, our children, or our finances.
1	2	3	4	5	My partner and I rarely make eye contact with each other.
1	2	3	4	5	My partner and I seldom laugh together.
1	2	3	4	5	I can't remember the last time my partner and I went out on a "date."

■ BTS 40

1	2	3	4	5	My partner and I disagree about the "right" amount of sexual activity.
1	2	3	4	5	My partner and I frequently have arguments about sex.

1	2	3	4	5	When we have sex, one of us is usually motivated by feelings of guilt.
1	2	3	4	5	When we have sex, one of usually ends up feeling resentful or "used."
1	2	3	4	5	In our relationship, the same partner usually initiates lovemaking.

Barriers to Sexuality
Phase VIII (Men and Women)

■ BTS 41

1	2	3	4	5	In terms of our relationship, I feel that my partner and I are not equally committed.
1	2	3	4	5	One of us contributes more to our relationship than the other.
1	2	3	4	5	My partner fails to keep his/her promises to me.
1	2	3	4	5	I do not think that my partner and I will be together in five years.
1	2	3	4	5	When we are angry with each other, my partner and I discuss ending our relationship.

■ BTS 42

1	2	3	4	5	I feel that my partner does not value my contributions to our relationship.
1	2	3	4	5	I feel that my partner is taking advantage of me.
1	2	3	4	5	I feel that my partner does not value my feelings or opinions.
1	2	3	4	5	My partner does not respect my time and my obligations outside of our relationship.
1	2	3	4	5	My partner does not treat me with respect around other people.

■ BTS 43

1	2	3	4	5	My partner does not notice when he/she has hurt my feelings.
1	2	3	4	5	My partner gives me the "silent treatment" to punish me or to get even with me.
1	2	3	4	5	I feel that my partner expects me to read his/her mind.
1	2	3	4	5	I feel like I never know what is going on in my partner's life.
1	2	3	4	5	I feel that my partner doesn't listen to my concerns, ideas, and problems with genuine interest.

■ BTS 44

1	2	3	4	5	I feel that I cannot freely express my feelings to my partner.
1	2	3	4	5	I am afraid to be totally honest with my partner.
1	2	3	4	5	I feel that my partner might consider having an affair.
1	2	3	4	5	My partner isn't always honest with me.
1	2	3	4	5	I feel that my partner keeps secrets from me.

■ BTS 45

1	2	3	4	5	My partner and I usually sit apart from each other when we're at home together.
1	2	3	4	5	My partner and I do not hug each other every day.
1	2	3	4	5	My partner and I rarely hold hands when we're walking together.
1	2	3	4	5	My partner and I sleep in separate beds.
1	2	3	4	5	My partner and I seldom touch each other playfully or lovingly.

BARRIERS TO SEXUALITY SCORES

BTS Phase I:
Diseases and Disorders in Men and Women

The questions for BTS 1 through BTS 11 pertain to risk factors for the following diseases or disorders. While even a single "yes" answer to any one of the listed questions can increase your likelihood of having or developing the relevant disease or disorder, the more questions you answer in the affirmative, the greater your chances of having or developing the relevant disease or disorder. Be sure to discuss your findings and your concerns with your physician.

Each of these conditions has the potential to lower your sex drive. In Chapters 4-8, I explain how, and tell you the steps you can take to eliminate—or at least minimize—the impact.

BTS 1: Heart disease (See page 87.)

BTS 2: Diabetes (See page 89.)

BTS 3: High cholesterol (See page 91.)

BTS 4: Hypertension (high blood pressure) (See page 93.)

BTS 5: Hypothyroidism (low thyroid hormone) (See page 98.)

BTS 6: Hyperthyroidism (elevated thyroid hormone) (See page 98.)

BTS 7: Chronic fatigue syndrome (See page 99.)

BTS 8: Obstructive sleep apnea (See page 130.)

BTS 9: Medication side effects (See page 139.)

BTS 10: Urinary incontinence in women (See page 121.)

BTS 11: Benign prostatic hyperplasia (BPH) in men (See page 125.)

BTS Phase II:
Emotional Disorders in Men and Women

The questions for BTS 12 through BTS 14 will help you identify emotional disorders that may be interfering with your libido or sexual performance. The more positive responses you have, the greater the likelihood that you're suffering from an emotional disorder. If you feel that you are at risk for the following conditions, it is important to discuss your concerns with your doctor or a mental health professional.

BTS 12: Depression (See page 102.)

BTS 13: Chronic stress (See page 171.)

BTS 14: Poor body image (See page 180.)

BTS Phase III:
Hormonal Imbalance

Affirmative responses to the questions for BTS 15 through BTS 19 may point to a hormonal imbalance, but the final diagnosis will likely depend on the results of blood tests and a physical examination.

Women

BTS 15: Premenstrual syndrome (PMS) or Premenstrual dysphoric disorder (PMDD) (See page 105–109.)

BTS 16: Perimenopause (See page 112.)

BTS 17: Menopause (See page 115.)

BTS 18: Testosterone deficiency (See page 117.)

Men

BTS 19: Andropause (See page 135.)

BTS Phase IV: Lifestyle Issues

If you answered "yes" to any of the questions for BTS 19 through BTS 25, lifestyle issues could be at the root of your diminished desire or suboptimal sexual performance. While you should definitely involve your doctor in addressing alcohol dependency, you can usually conquer the other lifestyle issues on your own.

BTS 20: Alcohol dependency (See page 177.)

BTS 21: Poor physical conditioning (See page 193.)

BTS 22: Sleep deprivation (See page 167.)

BTS 23: Overwork syndrome (See page 12.)

BTS 24: Poor eating habits (See page 201.)

BTS 25: Poor nutritional balance (See page 201.)

BTS 26: Caffeine dependency (See page 179.)

BTS Phase V: Sexual Dysfunction

The questions for BTS 27 through 33 are designed to help you determine if a sexual dysfunction is at the root of diminished desire or performance problems. If you answered "yes" to one or more of the questions in this section, and you suspect that you have one of the following conditions, your physician will be able to confirm the diagnosis and recommend the appropriate treatments.

BTS 27: Hypoactive sexual desire disorder (HSDD) (See page 68.)

BTS 28: Orgasmic disorder (See page 82.)

Women

BTS 29: Female sexual arousal disorder (FSAD) (See page 79.)

BTS 30: Sexual Pain disorder (See page 76.)

BTS 31: Vaginismus (See page 78.)

Men

BTS 32: Premature ejaculation (See page 75.)

BTS 33: Erectile dysfunction (See page 71.)

Phase VI: Conversation Style

BTS 34: Right-brain conversationalist (See page 58.)

BTS 35: Left-brain conversationalist (See page 58.)

Phase VII: Sexuality Issues

BTS 36 through 40 will help you uncover sexuality issues that may needsome work. Add your scores for each BTS, and then use the following grading system:

Score	Evaluation
	Needs immediate attention
9-16	Needs improvement
17-25	Not a problem

BTS 36: Sexuality is not a priority

BTS 37: Sexual identity issues

BTS 38: Your sex life is in a rut

BTS 39: Intimacy deficit

BTS 40: Desire discrepancy (See Chapter 3.)

Phase VIII: Relationship Issues

BTS 41 through 45 will help you identify barriers to sexuality in your relationship. Use the same grading scale as above.

BTS 41: Commitment

BTS 42: Respect

BTS 43: Communication

BTS 44: Trust

BTS 45: Touch

HE WANTS "IT," SHE DOESN'T:

Here's Why

IT'S ONLY NATURAL FOR TWO PEOPLE TO HAVE DIFFERENT OPINIONS about what is and what isn't enough sex, especially when one of those people is a woman and the other is a man. This doesn't necessarily indicate that one partner is suffering from hypoactive sexual desire disorder. The problem could be simple "desire discrepancy," the single most common complaint heard by most sex therapists. In fact, in surveys among couples, men almost always say that they don't get enough sex, while women are more likely to say that they're getting more than they really need.

Debbie and Jeff are pretty typical in this respect.

"Jeff would have sex every day of the week if I'd agree to it," says Debbie. "I don't think that's normal. He doesn't understand that I just don't feel like having sex that often."

Jeff sees the situation differently: "Of course I want to have sex every day. Who doesn't? When two people are in love, it's normal to want to have sex as often as possible."

While Debbie and Jeff disagree about what constitutes a "normal" level of sexual desire and activity, there's really no such thing. Part of the reason for this rather large variance in sexual appetite between the genders is the biological makeup of the male and female brain and body. Debbie wishes that Jeff wouldn't want sex so much, but for Jeff, wanting sex may be more a result of his brain's innate "maleness" than his conscious thought. Men are driven to have sex more often than women because of higher testosterone levels, which, in the average man is about twenty times higher than that of the average woman. With so much of the hormone of desire coursing through their bodies and bathing their brains at any given time, sex is almost always on the male mind, and their bodies are almost always ready and willing to accommodate.

Jeff wishes that Debbie desired sex more often. Debbie, like most women, doesn't have the hormonal makeup to drive her to seek sex at every opportunity. Compared to men, women have relatively low levels of testosterone, and as a result, sex isn't always at the forefront of their minds.

I wish more couples understood this. When I explained this to Debbie and Jeff, it allowed them to be a little more understanding of each other's sexual appetites, and more considerate of each other's needs. I also recommended that they take advantage of Debbie's heightened levels of desire in the middle of her monthly cycle. Around the time of ovulation, when the woman is most fertile, her testosterone and estrogen levels peak. This may create a welcome surge of libido, driving her to seek out sexual activity.

If you and your partner experience the same kind of "desire discrepancy" as Jeff and Debbie, it may help both of you to pay more attention to the woman's menstrual cycle, and take advantage of this prime opportunity. For women with a twenty-eight day cycle, ovulation—and peak estrogen and testosterone levels—occurs between the twelfth and sixteenth days of the cycle, when day one coincides with the onset of menstrual bleeding.

Paying attention to this cycle worked well for Debbie and Jeff.

"I never really noticed it before, but that's the time of the month when I really feel like making love, and I'm not just doing it to please Jeff," says Debbie.

When Debbie allowed herself to follow her instincts during this phase of her cycle, she was able to engage in sex in a way that was deeply satisfying for Jeff. "I love it when I know that Debbie wants me," he said. "It's a huge turn-on." He confessed to me that he still would have liked to have sex more often, but this compromise helped.

THE FULFILLMENT FACTOR

Hormonal differences aren't the only factor contributing to the differences in male and female sexual appetites. Consider the fact that nature rewards sexually active men by virtually assuring them physical gratification through orgasm in every sexual encounter.

Women should be so lucky. Only about 20 percent of women routinely experience orgasm with sexual intercourse. What women typically want from their sexual encounters are affection and intimacy. They don't expect physical gratification—as men do—because sex may not always provide them with consistent physical fulfillment.

This was the issue for Renee and Dustin. They both enjoy sex, but when they came to me, Renee didn't want to make love as often as Dustin, primarily because she didn't find it all that satisfying.

"I think I would want to have sex more often if I enjoyed it more," she told me. "Sometimes I feel like Dustin is just using me. I wish he would slow down a little. Once we decide to make love, he practically pounces on me, and I feel like he forgets about me and what I need. By the time I'm just getting warmed up, it's over."

I helped her to understand that Dustin's brain and body are under the influence of testosterone, and therefore almost perpetually primed for sex. In addition, the male brain, which I'll discuss a little later, causes a man to be single-minded and goal-oriented. So when Dustin "practically pounces" and becomes seemingly self-absorbed, he's simply pursuing his goal, which is to achieve orgasm.

It was just as important for Dustin to understand—and become more attentive to—Renee's needs when they made love. When he learned how important foreplay was to Renee, he was more than happy to change his approach. Now, prior to making love, they spend more time touching. Dustin also pays more attention to stimulating Renee through longer periods of foreplay. This made a big difference for both of them.

Once Dustin learned how to help Renee become more fully aroused, she found it easier to experience orgasm and a sense of physical fulfillment. As a result, she found herself wanting to have sex more often—which suited Dustin just fine.

While women need more physical stimulation than men in order to become sexually aroused, they also need more emotional stimulation. Because of the way a woman's brain is organized, women are able to experience intimacy in ways other than sexual activity. The emotional stimulation of having meaningful conversations can provide a gratifying dose of intimacy for most women. Fortunately, men can learn to take advantage of these pathways to pleasure.

Carl and Sarah had been married for seven years when their discrepancies in sexual desire began to create problems in their relationship.

"Carl expects me to just jump into bed with him at a moment's notice," Sarah told me. "He gets turned on at the drop of a hat, and he thinks that I should, too. He doesn't realize that I need to be romanced a little first." For Sarah, as for most women, the "goal" of lovemaking is usually the opportunity to revel in the relationship and enjoy the intimacy that it brings.

While men are more sensitive to visual stimulation, women are more receptive to tactile and auditory stimulation. This means that women like to be touched in a loving manner, and like to engage in a little loving conversation. While just looking at his lover may be a real turn-on for a man, this usually isn't enough for a woman, no matter how attractive her mate may be.

Carl was willing to do just about anything to reignite Sarah's desire for sex. He agreed to spend more time and effort romancing her. He found that when he started cuddling and conversing with Sarah, she not only agreed to have sex more often, but she actually began to initiate lovemaking.

To women, asking a male lover to just talk or open up seems like a very small matter. But it's important to appreciate the fact that this doesn't come naturally to men—in fact, it's often rather difficult. That's because their compartmentalized brains are better equipped to deal with problems, spaces, and objects than they are with words and language. Furthermore, the "emotional" areas of their brains are only loosely connected to the "talking" areas of their brains, and they often have a great deal of difficulty putting their emotions into words.

For men, the goal of speech is to communicate information or to solve a problem. For women, it is a way to share feelings and establish intimacy. When a woman wants to talk about a problem, she often feels hurt and misunderstood when her male partner tersely delivers a verbal solution. While the woman may be left feeling that her mate isn't listening or doesn't care, it's probably not the case. The action-oriented man doesn't share or understand her need to "talk things out," and he thinks he's being most helpful by figuring out how to solve the problem. Many men have trouble talking just for the sake of making conversation, and women need to be appreciative and understanding of their valiant efforts.

WHEN MEN EXPERIENCE LOW LIBIDO

When desire discrepancies crop up in a relationship, it is almost always an issue of the man wanting more and the woman wanting less sexual contact. When men experience low libido, it is typically a result of emotional issues, hormonal imbalances, or illness. Depression, anxiety, low testosterone levels, and heart disease can dramatically diminish sexual desire in men. Occasionally, even healthy, well-adjusted men will experience diminished sexual desire. A man may apply his single-minded focus to some other aspect of his life that he deems equally as important as sex, like providing for his family. John, a thirty-eight-year-old real estate agent, found himself in this situation.

"It's tough to make a living in real estate right now," he explained. "The market is down, and people just aren't buying houses like they were two years ago. I'm working twice as hard to make the same income."

Carol appreciated the fact that John was working hard, but she felt neglected. "He acts like he doesn't want to be with me. Even when we're alone and we have a chance to make love, he's at his desk, making phone calls." While John may feel as if he's sacrificing his own needs to support his family, Carol feels as if he's sacrificing their relationship.

In addition to the very real, innate discrepancies in the male and female brains, and perhaps because of them, there are plenty of other reasons why men and women have different sex drives. Stress and fatigue are two such reasons. For working women and women with children, stress and fatigue have become a way of life. The deeply embedded maternal instincts of a woman drive her to satisfy the needs of her children before addressing those of her mate. Because people and relationships are so important to her, she may feel compelled to attend to others, even at her own expense. When she's feeling overworked and overwhelmed, sexual activity often gets put on the back burner.

Andrea, a social worker and mother of two young children, is the perfect example.

"I get up at the crack of dawn, knowing that I have a thousand things to do," she said. "I get the girls ready for school, and get myself ready for work. I make breakfast and pack lunches. I go to work for nine hours, and I deal with a hundred people and their problems. After work, I pick up the girls from the babysitter's, and the minute we get home, I have to make supper, wash clothes, and help the girls with their homework. Roger helps out, but when it's all said and done, it's really up to me. When I finally tuck the girls into bed around nine o'clock, I'm literally exhausted. That's usually when Roger wants to make love. When he starts rubbing my back—that's his way of coming onto me—I could just *scream*! Why can't he understand that I'm dead tired, and I just don't have anything left to give?"

Given Andrea's hectic lifestyle, it's understandable that she was stressed out and tired. As a woman, her brain is geared to make sure that her children, her home, and her relationships are well cared for, and these things naturally take precedence over sexual activity. As a human being, however, she has physical and emotional limits. She can do only so much before her mind and her body, not to mention her sexual energy, begin to suffer.

Roger, Andrea's husband, told me he admires the way she juggles work and family responsibilities. "She's very good at what she does, and she's a great mother to our girls," he said. "But sometimes, I wish she'd just let the laundry sit for an evening and make love to me." Like most men, Roger feels that sex is infinitely more important than housework.

WHAT TO DO WHEN YOU'RE NOT IN THE MOOD

Should you have sex to please your partner even when you're not in the mood? This is the million-dollar question, and the right answer may depend on the intensity of your feelings, your partner's feelings, and the situation at hand. Whether you reluctantly choose to have sex with your partner or decide to abstain, one of you will undoubtedly end up being unhappy with your decision.

The question of whether or not to have sex when you're not feeling up to it is one that has perplexed me since I began my career as a physician. As part of my medical training, I worked in a rural health clinic for women in a remote part of southwestern Virginia. One of my first patients was a young woman, who was accompanied by her three small children. When I asked her how I could help her, she told me that her husband had brought her to the clinic to find out what was wrong with her. When I asked her what sort of problem she was having, she replied, "I don't want to have sex no more." She went on to say that she feared that if she didn't start satisfying her husband's needs, he would "get it somewhere else."

In trying to better understand the situation, I gently asked, "Are you still sexually active, even though you don't feel like it?" The young lady immediately replied, "Oh no, I ain't active. I just lay there."

In my youth and inexperience, I was dumbfounded that the act of lovemaking between married adults could be reduced to something as tragically base as "just lying there." Now that I have a few years of experience as a physician under my belt, I'm no longer surprised when

I hear people describe their feelings and actions in similar ways. Even though they may not use the same terminology as the young woman from Virginia, it is often just a variation of the theme. Not infrequently, I hear phrases like, "I just go through the motions," or "I only do it because I feel like I have to," or "I just grit my teeth and wait for it to be over."

The question of whether or not to have sex with your partner when you're in a committed relationship, even when you don't feel like it, is one that just doesn't have a right answer. To engage in sexual activity against your wishes seems like a violation of your human rights. After all, it's your body, and you should be able to decide what you will do or have done to it. On the other hand, when you're involved in a monogamous relationship, it becomes a game of *Tag! You're it.* Your partner has nowhere else to turn. If your partner truly wants and needs sexual contact to feel fulfilled as a human being, remaining unwillingly abstinent for long periods of time seems like a violation of his or her human rights.

If you're struggling with the question of whether or not to make love to your partner even when you don't feel like it, your best bet may be to simply change the question. Ask yourself this: What would it take to put me in the mood to make love? You may not know the answer at this point, but the good news is that there is definitely a right answer— or even several right answers—to this question. This book may help you find them.

HMM, SEX TONIGHT OR THE LAUNDRY?

The highly integrated brains of women make them champion multi-taskers. They're acutely aware of the dozens of things that must be done every day to keep their lives running fairly smoothly. When it comes to sexuality, being a multi-tasker can be a curse. For the woman with a million things on her "to do" list, it can make just "being" extremely difficult. Many busy women find it hard to adopt the focused, single-minded pursuit of sexual enjoyment as effortlessly as men do.

Men can help free their female partners from the chains of their multi-tasking brains by offering to help them. Simply asking, "What can I do to help you out?" goes a long way toward lightening the load.

Nancy, a forty-two-year-old attorney and the mother of three teenagers, says that for her, this is the equivalent of foreplay. "When Bob notices that I'm getting overwhelmed, he always comes to my rescue. He'll offer to make dinner for the kids, or do the laundry for a week. He doesn't know it, but that's the biggest turn-on there is."

Women, on the other hand, need to accept the fact that no matter how stressful or busy their lives become, it's critical to take the time to address their husbands' innate and almost irrepressible sexual needs. If women understood how central a man's sexuality is to his sense of self, his self-esteem, and his very being, they'd likely give it a higher priority in their schedules and in their lives.

When my female patients tell me about the problems in their relationships that are caused by desire discrepancies, it's very easy for me to sympathize with them. I see how hard they're working to stay on top of their incredibly busy lives. Many of them have demanding jobs, aging parents, and active young children. They feel as if they're being pulled in a dozen different directions. It seems perfectly understandable that their sexuality might take a back-seat to what seems like their daily survival.

On the other hand, my heart also aches for many of my male patients who are suffering the emotionally devastating consequences of desire discrepancies. They often feel totally rejected, unloved, and unworthy. Emmett, a professional baseball player, explained these feelings to me:

"I came home for a three-day break after being out on the road for over six weeks," he said. "I was so happy to see my wife, and I couldn't wait to be with her. I couldn't believe that she didn't want to make love to me." Although Emmett's wife may have wanted more time to reconnect and reestablish intimacy, to Emmett it felt like a slap in the face and a total rejection of his love. For most men, sexual rejection is an incredibly painful experience.

Repeatedly ignoring or denying your male partner's sexual needs may cause him to question his self worth. Joel told me about his self doubt:

"My wife hates having sex with me," he said. "I can't remember the last time she even slept with me. When she puts the kids to bed at night, she just stays there with them. I wonder what it is that's so wrong with me? What is it about me that's so bad that she won't even sleep with me?"

Joel's feelings aren't at all uncommon among men who are sexually unfulfilled. Studies have shown that men who remain involuntarily celibate for long periods of time are likely to suffer from feelings of anger, depression, and worthlessness.

Not acknowledging or fulfilling your male partner's sexual needs may also lead him to consider the alternatives. Darrell, a forty-four-year-old CEO of a major manufacturing company confided in me that he's struggling with a decision that may tear his family apart.

"I love my wife more than anything in this world. Of course I love my kids, but I love their mother even more," he told me. "I want to make love to her, but she never wants to anymore. It's not just about the sex—I really wish my wife wanted me like I want her. I need my wife's love, and she just doesn't seem to feel it for me. I'm wondering if I should spend the rest of my life in a relationship with a woman who doesn't really love me." At some level, Darrell's wife may realize that she's not fully satisfying his sexual needs, but I doubt if she understands that her sexual withdrawal has left him feeling so unloved that he's considering leaving her.

Like Darrell, Jared is examining his options.

"My wife hasn't made love to me in over six months," he told me. "Before that, I think we went four months without having sex. The way I see it, I've got two choices. I can keep on being a good and faithful husband, and accept the fact that I'm going to be practically celibate for the rest of my life. Or I can leave my wife and have all the sex I want. But that would make me a major jerk, and that's just not who I am."

When Jerome talked about what he perceived as his wife's rejection, he couldn't hide his bitterness. "I'm not a bad-looking guy—plenty of women hit on me. But having sex with my wife is like pulling teeth. I'm lucky if I get it once a month. I just think it's pretty ironic. Here I am, a decent looking, reasonably successful guy, and I'm in the bathroom jerking off in my own house, because my wife can't stand for me to touch her."

While men may talk more about the rejection of their sexual advances, what they're feeling is a rejection of their love. The message that I hear over and over from men who feel that their wives aren't fulfilling their sexual needs is this: "I just want to feel needed. I want my wife to want me. I want to know that I'm her man." Even if your male partner complains to you about his lack of sexual fulfillment, what he really means is that he feels rejected. He wants your acceptance and approval. He wants to know that he's the only man for you, and that you need him as much as he needs you.

If your male partner lets you know that he's feeling hurt, lonely, or neglected because he misses making love to you, you can bet that it is incredibly important to him. If it's bothering him enough that he wants to talk about it—something that doesn't come easily to him—he's undoubtedly suffering a great deal. If your mate isn't able to fully express those emotions in words, he may be doing what comes more naturally to men. He may be clamming up, surrounding himself with space, and distancing himself emotionally. Unfortunately, these tactics usually only make matters worse, and often lead to a stand-off in the relationship.

When it comes to your most treasured relationship, it is always more important to do the right thing, rather than to just be right. Try reaching out to each other, and show your partner your love by giving of yourself both emotionally and physically. You'll probably be amazed to find that once your partner feels loved, understood, and accepted by you, he or she will be in a better position to return love in ways that are most satisfying to you.

HOW GENDER-RELATED DIFFERENCES FUEL FIGHTS ABOUT SEX

Although every individual is unique and every couple is different, some trends and traits seem so distinctly gender-specific that it's fairly safe to make some generalizations. Perhaps you and/or your partner are the exceptions. Broadly speaking, however, when it comes to physical, biological, and hormonal makeup, women are typically more like each other than they are like men, and the reverse is also true. In fact, the difference between the sexes reaches down to the cellular level. Why should it be any surprise that their behaviors are different as well? They are very different, despite the efforts of psychologists, sex therapists, and scientists to bend their findings and opinions to satisfy the gods of political correctness and gender equality.

These physical and hormonal differences color sexual appetites, attitudes, and expression. Thus, they wield considerable influence in love and sexual relationships. To understand the discrepancies in sexual desire between men and women, you need to understand why they exist.

Differences in Socialization

For the past several decades, perhaps in acquiescence to the women's movement, it has been fashionable to try to explain away the very real differences between the sexes by pointing to discrepancies in societal conditioning. Boys are raised to be tough and aggressive, while girls are taught to be caring and cooperative. Boys are encouraged to conquer, compete, and build with toy guns, games, and erector sets, while girls are given dolls and tea sets, the better to hone their domestic and maternal skills.

It has been argued that infants are born sexually neutral, and would likely continue to develop in a type of genderless sameness, if not for the sexist interventions of parents, teachers, and society in general. The politically correct dogma was that biology had less to do with our "maleness" and "femaleness" than the culture in which we were raised, and society was held accountable for the vast majority of the differences between the sexes.

Although these theories prevailed for years, they are now being soundly and consistently overturned. Modern technology and scientific discovery have allowed us to peer more closely into the brains of men and women, and to gain a greater understanding of the ways in which they work. What we have found is that they are markedly different in terms of organization and function.

It is impossible to separate our natural traits from those that were formed as a response to societal expectations and cultural pressures. But given the distinct contrasts in the biological makeup of men and women, it is naïve to think that social conditioning alone is responsible for all of the ways in which men and women differ. While the environments in which we are raised may reinforce these differences, many of them exist even before we are born.

Hormonal Differences

To a large degree, our hormones are responsible for stereotypical male and female behaviors. The ways in which we act and think are governed to some extent by the levels of hormones coursing through our veins: namely, estrogen in women and testosterone in men. These hormones determine the distinct male or female organization of the fetal brain.

Although gender is determined at the time of conception, it isn't until about the sixth week of embryonic development that a distinct gender emerges, when the specialized cells in the male fetus begin to produce male hormones, primarily testosterone. These hormones lead to the development of male genitalia. In the absence of male hormones, the fetus will develop female sexual organs.

In the uterus, the male fetus is exposed to high levels of testosterone at the precise time that its tiny brain is beginning to take shape. Exposure to the male hormone at this critical stage of development will determine the organization and future function of the brain. In short, it generates the male mind-set. In the absence of exposure to testosterone, the brain of the girl fetus will develop, resulting in the ultimate creation of the female mind-set.

Throughout infancy and childhood, boys and girls share the same types of hormones in roughly equal concentrations. Once puberty strikes, however, the hormonal makeup of adolescent boys and girls diverges dramatically. In boys, a massive surge of testosterone works to increase muscle mass, promote the growth of facial hair, and lower the voice. In girls, rising estrogen levels bring on menstruation, and lead to the redistribution of body fat, resulting in softer curves and rounder physiques. At the same time that these hormones are transforming the bodies of adolescent boys and girls, they are also exerting a powerful influence on their brains.

Brain Organization Differences

If hormonal influences alone were responsible for the profound differences in males and females, you would expect that little boys and little girls would behave similarly in childhood, when the hormonal makeup of the two genders is practically identical. Since this is obviously not the case, there must be another explanation.

The explanation lies in the fact that the brains of boys and girls—and later men and women—work quite differently. With the exposure to testosterone at a critical time in fetal development, the male brain undergoes transformations that do not occur in the female brain. These organizational variances lead to profound contrasts in the ways in which men and women think, feel, and act, and especially in the ways that they experience and express their sexuality.

Left Brain vs. Right Brain Preferences

Structurally, the brains of men and women are almost identical. By adulthood, the average human brain tips the scale at just under three pounds. In both sexes, the brain is divided neatly into two halves, the left and right hemispheres. The division of labor between these two mirror images is so striking that they behave almost as if they were two separate brains. How men and women use the two sides of the brain and the sum of their parts undoubtedly sets the stage for the sharp contrasts between them.

In general, males tend to rely more heavily on the right side of the brain, the half that specializes in handling visual and spatial problems. The right brain controls abstract thought processes, and is responsible for seeing the "big picture." As right-brainers, men tend to be especially skilled at tasks involving spatial reasoning, like map reading, and those involving mechanical skills, such as assembling or repairing a lawnmower.

Although women use both halves of their brains to a greater extent than do men, they typically rely more heavily on the left side, the hemisphere that governs language and verbal abilities. Left-brain dominance helps explain why girls learn to speak earlier than boys, and why women spend more time engaging in conversation than men.

As right brain thinkers, men tend to learn best when they are allowed to visualize. As left-brainers, most women learn more efficiently by hearing, rather than by seeing. In practical terms, hemispheric dominance may help answer the age-old question about why men seem almost incapable of asking others for directions, while women seem to have more trouble reading maps, and then refolding them when they're finished.

In men and women, the right and left hemispheres of the brain are connected by a structure called the corpus callosum, a massive bundle of nerves comprised of over two hundred million neural fibers. This sophisticated communication system functions as a living computer cable, coordinating the functions between the two halves of the brain. The greater the number of connections between the two hemispheres, the more articulate a person is. This helps provide an explanation for women's outstanding verbal dexterity and conversational skill. It is estimated that a woman's corpus callosum—on average—is 23 percent larger than a man's.

The high degree of communication between the two halves of the brain contributes to a woman's ability to do several things at once, earning her the reputation of being a "multi-tasker." By allowing a woman to coordinate facts and feelings so efficiently, it undoubtedly accounts for her uniquely perceptive intuition. Men's brains, on the other hand, are more compartmentalized and specialized, allowing them to approach their work, play, and just about anything else with a single-minded focus, without being distracted by extraneous information. Because their brains keep facts and feelings in separate mental files, they're typically far less intuitive than women.

In men, emotions are generated primarily from the right side of the brain. Because men's brains are more compartmentalized, men are better able to keep their emotions in check, and to themselves. With emotional responses residing in the right half of the brain, and speech predominantly in the left half, men are less able to express their emotions in words. Because the two halves of the brain are connected by fewer fibers than a woman's, the flow of information connecting emotions and language is restricted.

Women, on the other hand, are less able to separate emotion from reason, and they're more likely to struggle to keep their emotions in check. In women, emotional responses are generated in both hemispheres of the brain. In addition, there is a greater exchange of information between the two sides of the brain, allowing the emotional side to be more fully integrated with the verbal side. Because what a woman feels is so effectively transmitted to the verbal side of her brain, she is quite adept at expressing her emotions in words.

In spite of the organizational and functional differences between the brains of males and females, it may still be tempting to think that some gender-specific behaviors are the result of environmental biases. After all, girls are encouraged to "talk about it," while boys are often given the message that "real men don't cry." But even before the influences of environment and culture have had a chance to mold and shape gender-specific behaviors, infant boys and girls behave in ways that are remarkably dissimilar.

While she is still in her mother's womb, the brain of the female fetus is organized to respond more acutely to all types of sensory stimulation. As children, girls place greater importance on people, relationships, and communication. When they are just a few hours old, girl babies are much more interested in people and faces, while boys routinely show greater fascination with objects like mobiles and rattles.

Newborn girls are more exquisitely sensitive to touch and sound than boys: They're also less tolerant of noise and pain. When they're upset, baby girls are more easily comforted by soothing words and singing than boys. Baby boys are more likely to respond to what they see than what they hear. Infant girls show greater interest in communicating, and they maintain eye contact with others almost twice as long as male infants. On average, newborn boys are much more active and spend less time sleeping than newborn girls.

Do parents unwittingly create these behaviors in their infant children? It's unlikely. Baby boys just naturally involve themselves in experiences that sharpen and refine their spatial skills, while baby girls involve themselves in experiences that enhance their interpersonal skills. As toddlers, boys want to explore objects and their surroundings because their brains predispose them to do so. Because girls' brains are better designed to talk and listen, they seek out opportunities that allow them to interact with others. Throughout childhood, boys remain more interested in objects and activities, whereas girls continue to show more interest in people.

How All These Differences Play Out in Love Relationships

The ways in which our brains are organized and influenced by our hormones dramatically affect how we think, communicate, and make love. Understanding the innate differences between your brain and your partner's can have a powerful impact on your sexual relationship.

Physically, men and women are generally attracted to each other because of their differences. Men prefer feminine physiques that are round where theirs are flat, that are soft where theirs are firm. Women prefer men who are taller than they are; and those with broad shoulders and narrow hips, in contrast to their own, fuller hips. Although most of us have no problem recognizing that we are attracted to members of the opposite sex because of their physical differences, many of us still expect our partners to behave, think, and feel in similar ways to ourselves. It's highly unlikely that we'll find both in the same partner. The very forces that create the desired physical features of the opposite sex are also responsible for the differences in their emotional makeup.

By design, a woman is more sensitive than a man. She is more aware of the nuances of touch, smell, and sound. The organization of her brain leads her to attach much more importance to the people and relationships in her life. In contrast, a man is more goal-oriented, more focused, and more single-minded in his approach to most areas of life, including his pursuit of sexual fulfillment. He is less sensitive to touch, and less acutely aware of the information provided by sound, which makes him less able to interpret the subtle nuances of language and conversation.

When it comes to sex, the differences between men and women become even more apparent, and often problematic. Even in relationships in which both partners share an enthusiasm for sex, the sexual appetite of the man almost always exceeds that of the woman. Sexual interest and awareness arrive earlier in boys and are almost always more important to them than to girls. Boys have erotic dreams far more often than girls, and can easily achieve orgasm through sexual fantasy, even in the absence of physical contact. Boys are typically more sexually active than girls. They masturbate more often, seek sexual gratification with greater gusto, and although they typically mature about two years later than girls, they tend to have sexual intercourse earlier and more often.

Before they commit themselves to a specific partner, men are more likely to be sexually promiscuous, with a greater number of sexual partners than women. Many men say that in the absence of true love, and without social and religious restrictions, they would continue to be happily promiscuous throughout their entire lives. Women, on the other hand, are much less interested in experimenting with a variety of partners. While men's sexual fantasies center on the sex act itself, women are more likely to fantasize about the romance that leads to love-making. While men are more interested in having sex, women are more interested in having relationships. Because of the organization of their brains, they often struggle to translate their emotions into words.

It's hard to imagine why the brains of men and women would be organized so differently as to seem impossibly incompatible. It's almost as if we are biologically set up to be forever at odds, and it's a wonder that any of us can make our love and sexual relationships work. Rather than bemoan these differences, it makes much more sense to acknowledge, accept, and even embrace them, since many of them are undoubtedly beyond our partners' control. To ask your partner to ignore or overcome his or her biological, hormonal, and cultural makeup is to ask the impossible.

This doesn't mean that you should give up trying to understand or be understood by your partner. It does mean that you shouldn't judge or criticize your partner for being who he or she is. It also means that you shouldn't waste a lot of time trying to change your partner, since it's unlikely to happen, and will only end up creating frustration and resentment. There will always be differences between you. Realize that it is these very differences that serve as the major force of attraction in your relationship.

CHAPTER 4

SEXUALITY AT ITS BEST

WHEN SEXUAL EXPRESSION FLOWS NATURALLY AND EFFORTLESSLY, one delightful phase triggers the exhilarating pleasures of the next, cumulating in a finale of ecstasy. The whole experience is capped off with a profound sense of sexual bliss.

When making love feels right, the act itself doesn't seem to be all that complicated. We just do what comes naturally, and the entire production seems less mechanical than mesmerizing. In reality, sexuality is an incredibly complex process involving both the mind and body. It is mediated by countless hormones, neurotransmitters, nerves, glands, and tissues. If our conscious efforts were required to coordinate the innumerable intricacies involved in the act of lovemaking, we'd probably never be able pull it off. Thankfully, our bodies and our minds are perfectly engineered for giving and receiving love through the act of sexual intercourse. As a result, most people are able to lose themselves completely in the act, and simply absorb the delightful sensations of the sexual experience.

Unfortunately, this isn't always the case. For various reasons, some individuals encounter obstacles in the expression of their sexuality. When sexual flow is interrupted, it is often necessary to take a step back, study the problem, and search for ways to overcome it.

As an individual, your sexuality is as unique as you are, encompassing the belief systems that have been imprinted upon you by your family, society, and religious institutions. On a conscious level, you may not like or agree with the sexual messages you received in your youth. You may not even remember them. Still, they can stagnate in your subconscious mind for years. When something happens to stir them, they come bubbling to the surface, and they may cause you some serious grief.

You know from experience that nothing in life is certain but change, and your sexuality is not immune to it. Sometimes, just when you seem to be getting the hang of it all, something in your life shifts, and you may find yourself engaged in yet another search for your true sexual self. Sexuality changes dramatically with the seasons of life. Age, maturity, and the wisdom gleaned from personal experience all work to smooth and polish your sexuality, creating a sexual identity that is as unique as your fingerprint. If that was all there was to it, the whole concept of sexuality would be a lot simpler. In reality, our sexuality is experienced in the context of our relationship with another individual. Each partner brings a special blend of sexuality to the relationship, each imparting his or her beliefs, attitudes, and responses to the act of making love. Undoubtedly, you have already stumbled onto the fact that there are dozens of potential trouble spots in this type of arrangement, and you have to stay on your toes to avoid them. In spite of your best efforts, sometimes a breakdown in one of these areas can occur, and the result can be sexual dysfunction.

THE SEXUAL RESPONSE CYCLE

The sexual response cycle is a model commonly used by physicians, scientists, and sex therapists to describe the changes that occur in the human body as a person engages in the act of making love. While the individual nuances of the sexual response cycle vary, most men and women can count on their bodies to tag all of the necessary bases in a set of well-defined steps that comprise the sexual response cycle. Although the current model of the sexual response cycle remains a work in progress, it is helpful to understand what *is* known at this point, with the goal of increasing our own sexual self-awareness.

In the 1950s, sex pioneers William Masters and Virginia Johnson put forth a model of the human sexual response cycle that was adopted almost unanimously and universally. After years of intense research, Masters and Johnson observed a common pattern of physical changes that occurred in men and women during the act of lovemaking. They identified four separate and distinct physical states achieved by the human body: arousal, plateau, orgasm, and resolution. Using the Masters and Johnson model, the sexual response cycle can be summed up like this: When men or women engage in lovemaking, sexual arousal progressively increases, leading to a plateau, at which no further arousal is possible, or necessary. Orgasm inevitably follows at the peak of the cycle, releasing sexual tension, and leading to a stage of profound physical and psychological contentment and relaxation, called resolution.

This Masters and Johnson model reigned until the late 1970s, when sex therapist Helen Singer Kaplan justifiably argued that it lacked an essential element: sexual desire. She proposed a three-stage model of sexual response that included desire, excitement, and orgasm. Many enlightened professionals embraced the idea that desire is indeed a critical component of the sexual response cycle. To ignore this issue is to assume that men and women are in a perpetual state of sexual readiness, regardless of the circumstances in which they find themselves. Teenage boys aside, most of us know that this is most definitely not the case.

Willingness

Sex expert Jo Ann Loulan offers possibly the most complete model of the sexual response cycle, with the notable inclusion of "willingness" as an important initial component of the process. She describes this stage as an "openness or receptivity to sexual stimulation." When you think about it, willingness is just as important as the other stages, and has earned its rightful place in the current model of the sexual response cycle.

Desire

Desire is the conscious wish to engage in sexual activity. Depending on the sensitivities of the individual, it may be triggered by sensual thoughts, visual, or auditory cues, or physical touch. Desire begins in the mind of the individual, and is thought to trigger a cascade of hormonal, biological, and neurochemical changes throughout the body. These changes begin gearing up the body for the experience of sexual activity.

Arousal

While the stages of willingness and desire have a decidedly intellectual element, arousal is the stage at which the body becomes involved. Arousal is the physical state of sexual excitement, triggered by dozens of changes in hormones, neurotransmitters, and nervous impulses. During this stage, blood rushes to the genital area, producing erection in men and vaginal engorgement in women. In women, the clitoris enlarges, the labia swell, and vaginal secretions become more copious. The nipples become erect as their sensitivity is enhanced.

Dilation of the blood vessels in the skin of the chest and breasts imparts a "sexual flush" that is commonly experienced by men and women during lovemaking. Depending on the person, the partner, and the level of passion, the arousal phase can last anywhere from a few short moments to several hours.

Plateau

In the plateau phase of the sexual response cycle, the pulse continues to quicken, breathing becomes more labored, and muscle tension increases. The sexual flush intensifies and spreads. In men, erections may grow momentarily harder, and in women, the outer third of the vagina may become even more engorged.

Sexual tension continues to build, bringing with it the awareness that orgasm is imminent and inevitable. The plateau phase is typically rather brief, lasting from around two seconds to a few minutes. With practice and experience, some individuals find that they are able to prolong this period, creating a more intense orgasm.

Orgasm

Orgasm is the climax of sexual excitement. Unfortunately, it is also the shortest phase, typically lasting for only a few exhilarating seconds. In general, women don't achieve orgasm as dependably as men. Perhaps by way of compensation, the female orgasm tends to last slightly longer that of her male partner, resulting in the rhythmic contractions of the uterus and the muscles surrounding the vagina. In healthy men, orgasm normally results in ejaculation, a process that serves to propel semen through the penis. Like women, men experience increased muscle tension throughout the body and rhythmic contractions of the pelvic muscles, an experience that people of both genders often describe in terms of "waves of pleasure."

Resolution

Following orgasm, the stage called resolution brings about a profound sense of physical relaxation, contentedness, and emotional well-being, often referred to as a state of "sexual bliss." For a moment or two, in the afterglow of lovemaking, all seems right with the world. During resolution, the body slows down, gradually returning to its former state.

The length of the resolution phase is longer in men than women. For a variable span of time, known as the "refractory" period, men are physically unable to achieve either erection or orgasm. Depending on health, age, and other factors, this stage may last for a period of minutes to days. As a rule, women are physically capable of responding to additional sexual stimulation almost immediately after an orgasm, although they may not wish to do so.

SEXUAL DISORDERS

According to the classification system used by the American Psychiatric Association, there are a dozen or so sexual disorders, divided into two main categories: *sexual paraphilias* and *sexual dysfunctions*. Sexual paraphilias tend to involve rather deviant or downright criminal behavior, and these fall far beyond the scope of this book. We'll stick to the sexual dysfunctions, which most commonly affect sexuality in terms of relationships.

Sexual Dysfunction

Sexual dysfunction is defined as any problem that interferes with the ability to engage in sexual activity. Sexual dysfunction can be subdivided into disorders that affect desire, arousal, and orgasm, as well as sexual pain disorders. Attention to male sexual dysfunction centers primarily around disorders of arousal, most notably erectile dysfunction. In spite of the narrow lens with which male sexual dysfunction is commonly viewed, men can also experience sexual dysfunction in terms of desire, orgasm, and sexual pain.

Sexual dysfunction in women is typically experienced and addressed much more broadly, and it is well-recognized that women are susceptible to problems in areas other than sexual arousal. Like men, woman can also experience dysfunction in terms of desire, orgasm, and sexual pain. Recent studies have found that in the general population, nearly 50 percent of women suffer some type of sexual dysfunction. Women have even earned their own, gender-specific category name: female sexual dysfunction.

As they relate to sexual dysfunction, the current terminology and classification systems can be quite confusing, even to the professionals who are involved in their diagnosis and treatment. If you suffer any type of problem related to your sexuality, finding a solution to the problem is much more important than deciding what to call it. With that in mind, it is still helpful to understand the various terms used to describe the conditions that can interfere with sexuality and the realization of sexual fulfillment.

Hypoactive Sexual Desire Disorder

Often referred to as low libido, HSDD is one of the most common problems associated with human sexuality. As defined by the American Psychiatric Association, hypoactive sexual desire disorder is the persistent or recurrent deficiency (or total absence) of sexual fantasies, thoughts, and/or desire for sexual activity, so much so it that causes personal distress to the individual.

When contemplating the diagnosis of HSDD, it is important to remember that there is really no such thing as a normal libido or a standard level of desire. Some people like to have sex on a daily basis, while others prefer it once a month. Since there is no gold standard with which to compare yourself, qualifying for the diagnosis of HSDD depends largely on your perception of your level of desire, and whether or not it is causing personal distress or difficulty in your relationship.

Hypoactive sexual desire disorder can be a problem that plagues certain individuals throughout their adult lives, or one that is acquired somewhere along the way. It can be generalized, meaning that it applies to every circumstance, or situational, in which it occurs with certain partners or in certain circumstances. It can have a single cause or multiple ones.

If you've ever worried that your libido might be a little lackluster, you're in very good company. Of the 43 percent of American women suffering from any type of sexual dysfunction, lack of desire for physical intimacy is the most common sexual complaint. Without a doubt, low libido is the most frequent concern voiced at sex therapy clinics. Several nationwide studies have shown that one in three women experiences a problematic loss of desire at some point in life. Although HSDD is more prevalent in women, the condition isn't totally unheard of in men: One in five men reports having experienced some degree of distress regarding low libido.

Since the source of the problem is often difficult to pinpoint, it can also be quite challenging to treat. Despite the degree of concern it causes, sexual desire, and female sexual desire in particular, remains a part of human sexuality that is not well-understood. It isn't uncommon for women with HSDD to have accompanying difficulties with sexual arousal or the ability to achieve orgasm, but this isn't universally true. The physiology of desire, arousal, and orgasm are entirely different processes, and although they are related, they are not necessarily interdependent.

Women who suffer diminished desire often have perfectly normal sexual function; they just can't seem to bring themselves to initiate any type of sexual contact with their partners. In most cases, they don't even feel up to being on the receiving end.

Just as there are many patterns of sexual desire, there are many reasons for a person to experience a change in desire. Some factors are medical in nature. Because testosterone plays a starring role in female and male sexual desire, a testosterone deficiency can be at the root of the problem. Suboptimal testosterone levels can be related to aging, menopause, or andropause, and to other medical conditions.

For some women, hormonal changes during and after pregnancy can trigger a change in sexual desire. Emotional problems often bring on a lack of libido, with depression being the most common culprit. Hypoactive sexual desire disorder can follow a traumatic sexual experience, such as rape or painful sex. Often, its roots lie in childhood, arising as a result of sexual abuse or messages from family and religious institutions that sex is shameful or sinful. In some cases, HSDD may be triggered by another sexual dysfunction, such as sexual arousal disorder, which can lead to painful intercourse, and thus, a diminished desire for sexual activity.

Relationship problems often lie at the heart of HSDD. When problems exist in the relationship, one or both partners may not feel comfortable engaging in sexual activity until conflicts are resolved. Even in stable, comfortable relationships, HSDD may stem from habituation between partners. Some couples become so familiar that their love relationship takes on a sibling-like quality, a phenomenon that tends to douse any feelings of sexual desire.

Finally, certain medications are known for their libido-lowering side effects. Antidepressants and drugs used to control blood pressure are the most common ones. Excessive use of alcohol or other drugs can also be a contributing factor.

Treatment of HSDD

Successful treatment of HSDD often depends on identifying its cause. No matter how difficult it may seem, it is important for you to discuss your concerns about your sexual desire with your doctor. Since training in human sexuality in medical schools is notoriously lacking, most physicians aren't geared to take your sexuality into account when inquiring about your general state of health and happiness. If your doctor fails to bring up the issue of your sexuality, you may have to initiate the discussion yourself.

Although many physicians don't feel qualified or comfortable providing the type of counseling that you may need, most are more than happy to refer you to a professional who is qualified to help you. In the meantime, your physician will probably want to rule out any underlying medical causes for HSDD, such as heart disease, hormonal imbalances, or diabetes. You can probably expect to undergo a few blood tests, as well as a review of the drugs, herbs, and over-the-counter medicines that you are currently taking. If one of your medications appears to be responsible for the problem, your doctor may recommend discontinuing it, lowering the dose, or replacing it with one that yields fewer sexual side effects.

While your doctor is covering all the medical bases, a qualified sex therapist, counselor, or psychologist can help you work though some of the emotional and relationship problems. Depending on your situation, the therapist may want to work with you alone, or with both you and your partner.

Pharmacalogic Treatment of HSDD

Pharmacological treatments of HSDD are generally directed toward correcting the underlying cause of the problem, whether it is depression, diabetes, or perhaps some combination of factors. Depending on your symptoms, your blood levels of estrogen and testosterone, and your overall state of health, you may be a candidate for treatment with hormone replacement therapy. Very few drugs exist for the sole purpose of treating symptoms of HSDD. There are however, several medications designed to treat other medical conditions that have demonstrated ability to have a positive impact on sexual desire. While these drugs have gained FDA approval for use in the treatment of certain medical diseases or disorders, that approval rarely encompasses the treatment of low libido. As a result, only a small percentage of doctors feel comfortable prescribing these medications in an "off-label" manner for the treatment of HSDD.

Sexual Aversion Disorder

Far more serious than HSDD is sexual aversion disorder—a persistent, extreme aversion to virtually any type of sexual activity. When sexual intercourse is attempted, individuals with the condition may experience a very real fear that is sometimes accompanied by panic attacks. Although the disorder occasionally occurs in men, it is much more prevalent in women and it usually has its roots in trauma, either from rape or sexual abuse. A repressive family or rigid religious upbringing can contribute to the problem.

In affected individuals, sexual activity may reignite the sensations of pain experienced in the past, even though intercourse may no longer be physically painful. Occasionally, medications can help alleviate feelings of anxiety and abort the panic attacks that accompany sexual activity, but some sort of sex therapy is inevitably necessary, especially for those who have experienced sexual trauma. Behavioral therapy is often used with varying degrees of success. In this type of therapy, the individual is gradually exposed to sexual activity, beginning with simple, nonthreatening touches. As comfort level increases, sexual intercourse may be introduced, and hopefully, enjoyed.

DISORDERS THAT AFFECT MEN

Erectile Dysfunction

Thanks to recent research and the advent of the wonder drug Viagra, the medical community—and indeed the entire world—is acutely aware of the prevalence of erectile dysfunction and the impact that it has on the lives of men and their partners. Erectile dysfunction is a widespread problem, affecting more than half of all men worldwide over the age of fifty.

Prior to our recent era of commercially endorsed enlightenment, men with erection problems weren't exactly encouraged to speak up or seek help. Just three short decades ago, sex experts Masters and Johnson boldly stated that in more than 90 percent of men with impotence, psychological factors were the primary cause. Men were led to believe that the inability to achieve or maintain an erection was somehow the result of a personal shortcoming. Undoubtedly, countless suffering men were told that their condition was just all in their heads.

As it turns out, the Masters and Johnson assertion couldn't have been further from the truth. In the thirty years that have since passed, research has revealed that only about 10 percent of cases of ED are purely psychological in origin. Ninety percent of men with ED are now thought to have a physical or biological basis for the condition. In the process of debunking the myths surrounding male sexuality, the word "impotence" has been appropriately shelved. Such a pejorative term only seems to make a worrisome condition sound worse.

As men grow older, their chances of experiencing ED increase. Every study done to date has noted that the single most reliable predictor of ED is aging. Studies suggest that after the age of fifty, between twenty and 50 percent of men have some degree of ED, and the incidence increases in proportion to age. By the age of seventy, an estimated sixty to 70 percent of men have ED. Still, there does exist a vigorous population of men in their eighties and nineties who continue to achieve impressive erections and enjoy fulfilling sexual encounters. This encouraging realization makes it clear that there's a little more to ED than just growing old.

It's likely that ED becomes more prevalent with age because aging is almost universally associated with the accumulation of cardiac risk factors. These risk factors affect not only the circulation to the heart, but also to the sexual organs. Included among the risk factors for both heart disease and sexual dysfunction are obesity, diabetes, high cholesterol, and high blood pressure. Also implicated are dozens of medications and chronic illnesses. As with most other diseases and disorders, ED is influenced by lifestyle factors, including smoking, alcohol consumption, and stress.

Although men with ED tend to focus their concern on its impact on their sexual performance, doctors are more likely to worry about its implications for cardiovascular health. Erectile dysfunction isn't solely a sexual or quality-of-life issue: In many cases it reflects the presence of underlying risk factors for heart disease. As your doctor is working with you to help overcome ED, he may also be taking a closer look at your cardiovascular health.

A complete workup for the condition of ED will undoubtedly involve a blood test to determine levels of testosterone. Adequate testosterone is critical to the achievement of erection, and if your levels are low, you may qualify for testosterone replacement therapy. While a low testosterone level is a possible explanation for ED, it's not the most common one, and other factors are usually involved. One of the hallmarks of a low testosterone level is a noticeable decline in sexual desire. If you've got a rip-roaring libido, your doctor may not even bother to check your testosterone levels.

Diagnosis of ED depends on a thorough history and physical examination, as well as the appropriate laboratory studies. Blood tests indicated in a workup for ED include blood sugar and cholesterol levels, and in some cases, prostate specific antigen (PSA) and testosterone levels. You'll probably be asked to provide a urine sample for analysis. Occasionally, hidden infections of the urinary tract or prostate gland can be responsible for your symptoms.

Your doctor will want to make sure that your symptoms aren't caused by psychological issues, including anxiety, depression, or relationship problems. If these are determined to be major contributors, or even minor ones, you'll undoubtedly be advised to seek the help of a counselor or therapist.

No matter how reluctant you are to share your problems with someone you haven't met and may not even like at first, studies repeatedly confirm that counseling is a highly effective treatment for ED with psychological roots. If you've never had counseling, your preconceived notions about it might be way off-base, and it certainly can't hurt to give it a try.

Treatments for Erectile Dysfunction

Viagra. By now, almost everyone in America has heard about Viagra, a drug that has helped millions of men reclaim their sexuality. It is important to understand that the drug isn't an aphrodisiac or a hormone: Viagra works by increasing blood flow to the genitalia. Just taking the medication will not increase libido or even cause you to get an erection: You must first experience sexual desire.

In most healthy men, sexual desire leads to erection. In order to achieve erection, the arteries in the penis relax and widen, allowing more blood to flow into the organ. As blood flows in, it becomes firm and erect, and the veins that normally carry blood away from the penis are compressed, thus restricting the outward flow of blood. Because more blood is flowing in and less is flowing out, the state of erection is achieved and maintained, making sexual intercourse possible. In men whose erectile dysfunction occurs as the result of a physical problem, blood doesn't flow into the penis properly. Medications like Viagra can help by increasing that blood flow. In spite of its celebrity status, Viagra isn't for everyone. If you take medicines belonging to the nitrate family of drugs, including nitroglycerine for the treatment of chest pain or other cardiovascular disorders, Viagra is definitely not for you. The combination of the two drugs could cause your blood pressure to drop like a rock, often to an unsafe or even life-threatening level.

Viagra isn't successful in producing erections in all men, and for others it may generate intolerable side effects, including headaches, facial flushing, and stomach upset. Less commonly, blurred vision or sensitivity to light may occur. Even if you can't take Viagra, or find that it doesn't work well for you, you still have a few other options, one of which may provide the perfect solution.

Apomorphine hydrochloride sublingual. Apomorphine hydrochloride is the first in a new class of erectile dysfunction drugs that act on the brain rather than directly on the penis. Marketed in Europe for over a year under the trade name Uprima, it has been shown to produce erections in most men within twenty minutes. The drug is believed to work by activating dopamine receptors in the brain.

Speed of onset is one of the new drug's greatest advantages. Some men are able to achieve erection within just five minutes of slipping it under the tongue. In contrast, men with erectile dysfunction are advised to take Viagra about an hour before they plan to have sexual intercourse. Although the new drug can be taken up to three times a day, it is likely that most doctors will recommend using it twice a week or so.

While apomorphine is very effective in producing erections in men with erectile dysfunction, it doesn't enhance libido or the intensity of orgasm. The drug seems to be safe and well-tolerated, and isn't known to interact with other medications. The most common side effect is mild to moderate nausea, which seems to fade with repeated use.

Prostaglandins. Agents called prostaglandins are known to facilitate erection, and doctors have used them in various forms for years in the treatment of erectile dysfunction. The prostaglandin Alprostadil is available as a penile injection (Caverject) or as a suppository that is inserted into the urethra (Muse). Needless to say, it takes a little courage to stick a needle into the base of your own penis, but if you can manage it, the results are usually satisfactory. Side effects can include penile bruising, pain, or rash; prolonged erection; and headaches. The urethral suppository occasionally causes penile bleeding and pain, as well as vaginal itching and burning in the partner. Prostaglandins may not be suitable for men with hypertension, or those who are taking certain medications for the treatment of high blood pressure or heart disease.

Vacuum Constriction Devices. For some men, the use of a medical appliance known as a vacuum constriction device provides a perfect solution for ED. In a recent study designed to measure the effectiveness of the vacuum constriction device, ninety-nine men with ED were instructed in the proper use of the appliance. Just two months into the study, seventy-eight of the men reported that they were able to achieve erections sufficient for intercourse by using the device.

At the start of the study, each man was asked to rate his typical erection on a scale of zero to one hundred. A rating of zero was equivalent to no erection at all, and a rating of one hundred signified the best erection of his life. At the start of the study, the average typical "erection score" was 41.3. Just two months after being given the devices, the score jumped to an impressive eighty-six. In addition to improving the quality of erection, the men reported dramatic improvements in sexual satisfaction during the study.

While vacuum constriction devices can provide an effective short-term treatment for ED, they may also help improve the condition over the long haul. Previous studies have shown that some men can actually "graduate" from the device. This is undoubtedly due to the fact that the use of vacuum constriction devices leads to improved blood flow to the penis. As blood flow to the area increases, it seems to help generate the growth of tiny new blood vessels in the penis, increasing the likelihood that a man will be able to achieve spontaneous erections in the future. For men with ED, it makes good sense to make a vacuum constriction device part of your therapeutic armamentarium. Not only are they useful in providing quick fixes, they may also contribute to a long-term solution.

Premature Ejaculation

Premature ejaculation is one of the most common sexual complaints among younger men. In a recent survey of college students, 65 percent of the men reported having experienced premature ejaculation on at least one occasion.

Premature ejaculation is a very subjective complaint, defined primarily by a man's attitudes and expectations. There is no preordained time after which you have engaged in sexual activity that you "*should*" have an orgasm. It's not like anyone's standing around with a stopwatch, clocking your performance. The only way ejaculation can be "premature" is if it occurs before it is desired. This is reflected in its official definition: the onset of orgasm and ejaculation that occurs persistently or recurrently *before* it is desired. In some cases, it occurs sooner than a man and his partner would like.

Premature ejaculation is probably due to a combination of emotional and physical factors. The problem is common among adolescent boys and seems to be intensified by feelings that sex is shameful or sinful. Fear of being caught in the act, of impregnating the partner, of contracting a sexually transmitted disease may be at the root of the problem, and performance anxiety only intensifies it. At a subconscious level, these concerns may persist into adulthood, and they are often magnified by relationship problems. Although premature ejaculation rarely has an underlying physical cause, inflammation of the prostate gland or a disorder of the nervous system may be to blame.

While it seldom denotes a significant physical problem, premature ejaculation can cause big problems for couples. If a man consistently ejaculates before his partner reaches orgasm, she may develop feelings of dissatisfaction or resentment toward him.

Treatment for Ejaculatory Disorders

Fortunately, several effective treatments for premature ejaculation exist. Sometimes, treatment is as simple as wearing a condom. Condoms can sufficiently reduce the sensation of the penis, necessitating additional stimulation before orgasm can occur. For most men, small doses of antidepressants of the selective serotonin reuptake variety (SSRI) are usually helpful. These drugs are well-known for their side effect of delaying orgasm. In some men, this phenomenon can be problematic and annoying, but for those who experience premature ejaculation, it may provide a virtual cure. The drug is effective when taken on a daily basis, or even an hour or two prior to sexual intercourse.

Another treatment commonly used for premature ejaculation is the start-and-stop technique. It involves stimulating the penis, either manually or through intercourse, until the man experiences the feeling that orgasm is inevitable. At this point, he and his partner stop providing stimulation, and wait for twenty or thirty seconds before resuming activity. It's a good idea to try this technique with manual stimulation at first, then advance to intercourse as you grow more comfortable with it. Use of the stop-and-start technique is effective in prolonging orgasm in more than 95 percent of men, allowing them to delay ejaculation for five to ten minutes, or even longer. Occasionally, premature ejaculation is caused by serious underlying psychological problems, for which psychotherapy may be appropriate and helpful.

DISORDERS THAT AFFLICT WOMEN—PRIMARILY

Sexual Pain Disorders

As the most pleasurable activity known to humankind, making love should never hurt. Unfortunately, experiencing pain with sex is not all that uncommon. Painful intercourse can occur in men, but it is far more common in women. Physicians use the term "dyspareunia" to refer to genital or deep pelvic pain experienced during intercourse. In women, it has several sources. Pain during intercourse may occur during the very first attempt at lovemaking. In virginal women, a membranous fold of tissue, called the hymen, may partially or completely cover the entrance to the vagina. Upon penetration during the first sexual encounter, the hymen may be torn, resulting in varying degrees of pain. While this type of pain is understandable, it is far more difficult to pinpoint the source of discomfort in women who have had sex comfortably, and even enjoyably, for years afterwards. Occasionally, pain may be the result of vaginal yeast or bacterial infections. Without proper treatment, these infections can linger for months or longer, significantly reducing the enjoyment of sexual intercourse.

In some women, pain may be the result of allergies to certain ingredients in contraceptive foams and jellies, or to the latex in condoms and diaphragms. Occasionally, these allergies may arise after the first exposure to the offending substance, but more often, the allergies take much longer to develop.

Any condition that affects the pelvis can be a source of pain during intercourse, including endometriosis, uterine fibroids, and pelvic tumors. Surgery, including hysterectomy and tubal ligation, can occasionally lead to the formation of scar tissue in the pelvic area. These fibrous scar tissues, called adhesions, can cause pain when they are pulled and stretched during sexual intercourse.

Although men can experience pain with intercourse, dyspareunia is far less common in males than in females. In men, dyspareunia may be the result of an infection of the urinary tract; a sexually transmitted disease; or prostatitis, an inflammation of the prostate gland. Men with Peyronnie's disease have a curvature of the penis that can make erections and attempts at intercourse painful. Some men report experiencing pain with orgasm while taking certain antidepressant medications, including amoxapine, imipramine, and clomipramine.

Because dyspareunia can occasionally be a red flag for a more serious underlying disorder, you'll definitely want to discuss the problem with your doctor. Blood tests may be performed to search for the source of your pain. If you are a woman, you'll probably end up on the receiving end of a pelvic exam, and you may be asked to submit to a pelvic ultrasound or other diagnostic study. In some cases, exploratory surgery is necessary.

If, after an exhaustive search, there is no readily identifiable explanation for your pain, your doctor may want to explore the possibility of psychological causes. It isn't uncommon for women with dyspareunia to develop anxiety or fear relating to sexual intercourse. Anger or resentment toward a sexual partner is also a possibility that must be considered.

Treatment of Dyspareunia

If there is no underlying physical problem in need of repair, your doctor will probably try to provide you with a means to make sexual intercourse less painful. For women, vaginal lubricants are often recommended. Even with these, many physicians and therapists recommend devoting more time to foreplay to optimize genital engorgement and vaginal secretion. In some cases, trying a different position during lovemaking is helpful, especially one that involves less deep thrusting, or one that gives the woman more control over the degree of penetration.

For both men and women, pain with intercourse is as unnatural as it is unpleasant. It is critical that you tell your doctor about it, so that the underlying cause can be identified. You may end up being diagnosed with a condition that isn't easily remedied, but at least you'll have the peace of mind that comes with understanding and the reassurance of knowing that it isn't life threatening.

Vaginismus

Vaginismus is the painful, involuntary spasm or contraction of the muscles of the lower third of the vagina that prevents sexual penetration. It is thought to arise from a woman's unconscious desire to prevent penetration and avoid sexual intercourse. The condition is usually attributed to psychological factors, and it occurs primarily in women who have experienced painful intercourse or sexual trauma in the past. These women may unconsciously wish to avoid penetration in an effort to protect themselves from the anticipated pain.

In the absence of sexual trauma, there are other explanations for the problem. Vaginismus may be triggered by the fear of losing control, or the fear of becoming pregnant. Women who received repressive or negative messages about sexuality as children may develop a phobic reaction toward sexual intercourse. Because vaginismus typically has a significant psychological overlay, most women with the condition will benefit enormously from counseling. Since vaginismus understandably produces a great deal of partner concern and anxiety, sex therapists often work with both partners to facilitate treatment. It is important and reassuring for the partner to realize that the muscle spasms that occur with vaginismus aren't under a woman's conscious control. The condition isn't necessarily a reflection on the relationship or on the feelings that a woman has for her partner. Nonetheless, most therapists will recommend that all attempts at sexual intercourse be put on hold until therapy is completed.

A complete medical history and physical examination can often help rule out any underlying physical problems that might be responsible for vaginismus. In addition to counseling, doctors often recommend using a method of treatment called the "graduated dilation" technique. Vaginal devices called "dilators" are prescribed to help women become accustomed to penetration. The term "dilator" is an unfortunate misnomer; the devices don't physically stretch the vagina. Rather, they are used to help women learn to progressively relax the muscles of the vagina. Very small devices are used initially, and as the woman becomes more comfortable, they are replaced with slightly larger ones. Once a woman can tolerate the insertion of larger dilators without discomfort, she and her partner can progress to sexual intercourse.

For women who are comfortable using their own fingers as "dilators," therapy may actually be more effective. Initially using one finger, a woman progresses to the insertion of two and three fingers as she gradually learns to relax the muscles of her vagina. As she gains greater control over these muscles, she can begin to allow her partner to perform the exercise. Sometimes it is helpful to "bear down" while performing the exercise, because it is nearly impossible to bear down and contract the muscles surrounding the vagina at the same time.

In the treatment of vaginismus, Kegel exercises can also be helpful. These are pelvic exercises in which a woman alternately squeezes and relaxes the muscles surrounding the vagina, allowing her to develop a sense of control. Combined with graduated dilation therapy and counseling, successful treatment of vaginismus has been achieved in more than 90 percent of women with the disorder.

Female Sexual Arousal Disorder

In the broad scope of things, female sexual arousal disorder (FSAD) is comparable to erectile dysfunction. Both are problems relating to the arousal stage in the sexual response cycle, with the end result being a level of physical arousal that is insufficient to allow the individual to engage in satisfactory sexual intercourse. At this point, it is important to remember that in clinical terms, the word "arousal" has a very precise definition. Although in everyday language we may use the words "arousal" and "desire" interchangeably, they have entirely different meanings when it comes to describing problems associated with sexual dysfunction. While desire implies a wish to engage in sexual activity, arousal may have nothing at all to do with interest in sex. Rather, it has everything to do with the body's physical response to sexual stimulation.

Some women who desperately desire sex find that they are unable to reach a physical state of arousal. On the other hand, many women who do not experience the desire for sex, but participate in an effort to please their partners, are perfectly capable of experiencing a normal state of physical arousal.

The difference between desire and arousal is pretty straightforward in men. Men who *desire* to have sex move on to the *arousal* stage of the sexual response cycle, in which they normally produce an erection. This highly visible sign leaves little doubt about the man's physical state of arousal. Women, on the other hand, give fewer visible cues about their physical state of arousal. This lack of a "sign" is a source of some confusion, not only to the affected individuals, but also to their partners and the professionals who try to help them.

When a healthy woman experiences sexual desire, she typically advances to the arousal stage of the sexual response cycle. In this stage, she will normally experience clitoral and vaginal engorgement, accompanied by an increase in vaginal secretions. It is at this point that female sexual arousal disorder causes problems. For whatever reason, her body fails to produce the genital changes that are necessary for enjoyable intercourse.

Like other types of sexual dysfunction, FSAD may be related to stress, poor body image, relationship problems, and a history of sexual trauma. In younger women with FSAD, psychological issues are more likely to be at the root of the problem than physical ones. Most young, healthy women in the premenopausal years are physically capable of achieving the state of sexual arousal, but psychological issues can certainly interfere with the process. In the search for the source of FSAD, it is important to consider prescription and over-the-counter medications, especially those used in the treatment of allergy symptoms. Any medication that dries the mucous membranes of the upper respiratory tract can dry those of the vagina as well.

In older women, or in younger ones who have had their ovaries removed, a hormonal imbalance may be to blame. The physical changes associated with sexual arousal are mediated by estrogen and testosterone, and without these hormones, the physical changes are extremely difficult to achieve. Just as men with very low levels of testosterone find it difficult or impossible to get an erection, women with low levels of estrogen and testosterone may find it difficult or impossible to achieve the physical state of sexual arousal.

With the discovery that the majority of men with male sexual arousal dysfunction (manifested as erectile dysfunction) have underlying heart or vascular disease, interest in these factors as a cause for FSAD has grown. It is now generally well-accepted that women with FSAD have many of the same underlying risk factors that contribute to ED in men, including diabetes, cardiovascular disease, high blood pressure, and high cholesterol levels. Each of these conditions is known to contribute to hardening of the arteries, which in turn interferes with the flow of blood to the genitals. Without the appropriate blood flow, women are unable to achieve the physical changes that normally occur with sexual arousal, including vaginal secretion, clitoral enlargement, and vaginal engorgement.

The onset of cardiovascular risk factors, combined with the vaginal dryness of menopause, make FSAD a rather common condition in the menopausal years. As a result, older women tend to require greater and longer periods of stimulation to reach a level of arousal that came more easily in their younger years. With insufficient stimulation, the female body does not achieve the physical state of arousal. As a result, vaginal secretions are scant, and sexual intercourse may be uncomfortable or even painful.

Treatment for FSAD

If psychological issues are thought to contribute to FSAD, counseling and sex therapy may be beneficial. Since FSAD may be due to inadequate stimulation, paying more attention to stimulation during foreplay is often helpful. Stimulation doesn't have to be limited to touch; it can involve erotic messages provided to any one of the senses. Since anxiety can effectively shut down the changes that typically occur with arousal, it is often helpful to take a warm bath before intercourse, listen to soothing music, or use an herbal remedy that promotes relaxation.

In perimenopausal and postmenopausal women, vaginal dryness is an inherent component of arousal disorders. Using a sexual lubricant may be helpful, although mineral oil and vitamin E are acceptable alternatives. Treatment with hormonal replacement therapy may dramatically increase vaginal secretions, correcting the problem of FSAD in a large majority of menopausal women. Applying estrogen and testosterone creams to the area not only increases lubrication; it also stimulates the vagina to produce its own, natural secretions.

A few small studies have shown that by taking medications that enhance blood flow to the genitalia, women with FSAD are able to realize favorable improvements in their symptoms. Theoretically, at least, Viagra would be one of these treatments, but so far, the drug is only approved for the treatment of arousal disorders in men. Fortunately, there are dozens of herbal remedies known to enhance blood flow throughout the body, and one of these may provide women with an effective alternative to Viagra in the treatment of FSAD.

Clitoral Therapy Devices

The U.S. Food and Drug Administration recently gave the thumbs up to a new device that promises to help women who suffer from female sexual arousal disorder. The Eros clitoral therapy device, called Eros CTD for short, is a soft, hand-held cup and battery-powered vacuum unit. When positioned properly, the suction-action provided by the device helps dilate the blood vessels in the area, causing relaxation of smooth muscle tissue and engorging the clitoris with blood.

These actions mimic the changes that normally occur naturally in women during the sexual arousal stage of the sexual response cycle. While the Eros-CTD helps women achieve adequate lubrication and sensitivity for an orgasm, it doesn't guarantee one.

The makers of Eros-CTD recently studied the effectiveness of the device in twenty-five women, in which fifteen suffered severe arousal dysfunction and ten did not. Of the fifteen women with FSAD, all reported experiencing greater sensation, while twelve reported improvements in sexual satisfaction. Eleven of the fifteen women with FSAD noted improved lubrication, and seven reported a greater frequency of orgasm. In the ten women without FSAD, some, but not all, reported improvements in the same areas.

Orgasmic Disorders

Physiologically speaking, orgasms in women and men are remarkably similar, but there is a rather large discrepancy in the ease of attainment. There are men who seem unable to orgasm, but their numbers are very few. Anorgasmia is thought to occur in less than 1 percent of healthy, sexually active men. On the other hand, the female orgasm can be frustratingly elusive. While about 85 percent of women report being capable of having an orgasm, only about a third of women have experienced orgasm during sexual intercourse. About 5 to 10 percent of adult women in the U.S. report never having experienced orgasm by any means.

Fortunately, the condition of anorgasmia is quite responsive to a do-it-yourself type of therapy. Just learning more about your body and the physiological processes involved in the attainment of orgasm can make a big difference. In some instances, anorgasmia is the result of inadequate sexual stimulation, or the sexual inexperience of either one or both partners. Rarely, orgasmic disorders may have physical origins, including diabetes or heart disease. Several types of drugs are known to interfere with orgasmic capacity, including narcotics, anti-anxiety drugs, alcohol, sedatives, and some antidepressants. In some cases, it may be due to another sexual problem, like inhibited desire. Your doctor or counselor can work with you to tease these issues apart and decide on the treatment methods that are best for you.

Treatment focuses on maximizing stimulation and minimizing inhibitions. Kegel exercises can be helpful, as they give women a greater awareness and sense of control over the pelvic muscles involved in orgasm. With a little work and a willingness to try new techniques or positions, women who are capable of generating their own orgasms will probably be able to achieve an orgasm during sexual intercourse.

The understanding and involvement of your partner can make achieving orgasm with sexual intercourse much easier. If you know precisely the type of stimulation that you need, it's important for you to muster up the courage to tell your partner how to do it for you. It might even be better to *show* your partner.

It is important to realize that not all women are able to achieve orgasm with the thrusting action of intercourse alone. The indirect clitoral stimulation that occurs with sexual intercourse just doesn't cover all the bases. In the now famous studies conducted by sex expert Alfred Kinsey, only about 30 percent of women were found to regularly reach orgasm by penile-vaginal intercourse alone.

Fortunately, many women find making love extremely enjoyable and fulfilling even in the absence of orgasm. These women are more likely to enjoy the process, rather than strive for the big "O." For people who are simply pleasure-oriented, the sensual enjoyment and intimacy provided by lovemaking are ends in themselves, rather than simply means by which to achieve orgasm. There's a great deal of merit in an approach that involves focusing on enjoying the process, rather than on winning the prize.

If you are interested in expanding your orgasmic horizons, here are a few steps that will help:

- Know what you want. Some women may strive to gain better control over their ability to have an orgasm, whereas others are intent on experiencing multiple orgasms.
- Know your body: It is difficult to expect your partner to please you if you aren't sure exactly what that entails. Give yourself permission to examine your own body, both visually and tactilely. You may benefit enormously from an anatomy book and a handheld mirror. Explore the different types of stimulation that are most pleasurable to you.

- Transfer your knowledge to your partner. Once you know what you want and need to achieve an orgasm, speak up! If you can't seem find the words at first, then try showing your partner what to do. Together you can work on achieving orgasm.
- Use sensate focus exercises explained below to elevate your awareness, and your partner's awareness, of what type of touch, pressure, or stroke feels most pleasurable to you.

Treatments for Orgasmic Disorders

Kegel exercises, named for their creator, Los Angeles physician, Arnold Kegel, are enormously beneficial to the sexual health of both men and women. They keep the muscles of the pelvis firm and healthy and increase the ability to control them. Men can use the exercise to delay orgasm, so they are especially useful in the treatment of premature ejaculation. Women often find the exercises helpful in attaining or intensifying orgasm.

Kegel exercises are designed to strengthen a specific set of muscles in the pelvis, called the pubococcygeal (PC) muscles. The PC muscles are familiar to all of us—they're the ones most commonly used to stop the flow of urine in midstream. Here's how Kegel exercises work: Contract your PC muscles by clenching them as though you're stopping the flow of your urine. Squeeze! Try to hold this contraction for two to three seconds, then relax. That's all there is to it! Start strengthening your PC muscles by practicing ten or twenty squeezes at a time, once or twice a day, and then work your way up, increasing the number of repetitions and the frequency. You can work on strengthening your PC muscles with Kegel exercises just about any time or any place. As long as you put on your poker face while you're at it, no one will ever know what you're up to.

Sensate Focus

Sensate focus is a giving and receiving exercise. Partners take turns giving and receiving touch and pleasure, initially avoiding the breasts and genital areas. The goal is to reduce anxiety and introduce individuals to the mutual pleasure that can be derived from simple touching. In performing sensate focus exercises, the receiving partner places his or her hand over the giver's hand to show where touch should be applied and what it should be like. This exercise improves communication between lovers, and helps them discover the delightful sensations they can achieve through mutual, pleasurable touch.

■ PART II

CHAPTER 5

YOUR LIBIDO AND YOUR HEALTH:

Making the Link

HUMAN SEXUALITY, WITH ALL ITS MYSTERIES AND MIRACULOUS INTRICACIES, is sensitive to the most infinitesimal changes in the mind and body. Any condition that affects your emotional or physical health can potentially interfere with sexual desire, performance, and enjoyment. If you have a medically diagnosed condition and low libido, you may not have made the connection.

In this chapter, I will brief you on the potential impacts of specific health conditions. Where appropriate, I will also suggest ways to work with your condition to eliminate—or at least minimize—its impact on sexual functioning.

Let's start with the conditions that affect men *and* women. Feel free to skip down to the one that's relevant to you. In the next two chapters, I will cover issues of special relevance to women, and then those relevant to men.

HEART DISEASE

Although heart disease is often thought of as a man's disease, in reality, it is an equal opportunity condition. American women are far more likely to die from cardiovascular disease than from any other cause. Currently, heart disease is the leading killer of both men and women over the age of sixty five. Although the condition typically manifests itself in women roughly twelve to fifteen years later than it does in men, it makes up for its late arrival with a vengeance. In elderly women, the severity of heart disease accelerates dramatically with age, surpassing that of men by the time women reach their late seventies or early eighties.

Recently, heart disease has been shown to have a close connection with sexual dysfunction, including arousal disorders in women and erectile dysfunction in men. The American Heart Association is so confident that this connection exists that it recently advised physicians to consider erectile dysfunction an early warning sign of coronary artery disease. In most cases, cardiovascular disease is caused by the accumulation of cholesterol buildup, known as "plaques," in the coronary arteries that supply the heart muscle with blood. These plaque formations are rarely limited to the arteries supplying the heart: They're frequently found in other blood vessels, including those that supply blood to the penis in men, and to the vagina and clitoris in women. Since erection and engorgement can occur only when the appropriate genital blood vessels are properly filled, it makes sense that any individual with cardiovascular disease—diagnosed or not—is at great risk for sexual dysfunction.

Fortunately, modern science has developed a vast array of medicines, surgeries, and other interventions that allow people with mild to moderate heart disease to remain among the living, and often enjoy a very satisfactory quality of life. In people with very severe cardiovascular disease, survival tends to takes precedence over everything else, and sexuality and quality of life may suffer as a result. In the most advanced cases, heart disease can leave its victims so frail and physically de-conditioned that they're simply unable to muster up the energy to engage in any type of physical activity, including sexual intercourse. Fortunately, these cases are rather rare, and most people with heart disease are completely capable of desiring—and enjoying—the act of making love.

In spite of its relative safety, it isn't all that uncommon for folks with heart disease to refrain from lovemaking, usually out of fear that they'll aggravate their condition and die in the act. I tend to agree with one elderly gentleman who sheepishly observed: "It's probably not such a bad way to go." Even if you don't share the same sentiment, the facts speak for themselves.

Research shows that dying during intercourse, or even shortly thereafter, is actually extremely unusual. One study found that less than 1 percent of all heart attacks occur within two hours of lovemaking activities. The risk of a sex-induced heart attack is even lower among people who exercise on a regular basis.

As long as you're not planning to swing from the chandelier in a G-string, the amount of physical exertion required for normal sexual intercourse has been determined to be roughly equivalent to that required to climb a couple of flights of stairs. If you've had a heart attack, or if you've been diagnosed with any type of heart disease, be sure to ask your doctor about your physical capacity to enjoy sexual activity. After the appropriate recovery time and necessary treatment, your physician will probably give you the green light. That's all the permission you need to relax and enjoy yourself, your partner, and your sexuality.

DIABETES

Diabetes is one of the most common causes of sexual dysfunction in both genders, and it is currently the leading cause of erectile dysfunction in men. There are two types of diabetes, conveniently dubbed type one and type two. For people with type one diabetes, regular injections of insulin are critical to survival. Those with type two can usually maintain control of their disease with oral medications; and in some cases, exercise and dietary changes alone will do the trick.

In healthy people, the body transforms food in the diet into glucose, a sugar that supplies energy to the millions of cells throughout the body. In order to gain access to those cells, it must travel through the bloodstream on the coattails of insulin, a hormone that is manufactured by the pancreas. In people with diabetes, the body is unable to use insulin properly, or to create it in the first place. As a result, glucose is denied access into the body's cells, and instead accumulates in the bloodstream, often to dangerous levels. Over time, these high levels of blood sugar can cause damage to cells and tissues, as well as to the veins, arteries, and nerves leading to virtually every part of the body. The eyes, kidneys, heart, and genital organs are most commonly damaged by diabetes.

Type one diabetes occurs when the pancreas is rendered incapable of producing insulin, necessitating daily injections of a synthetic form of the hormone. This type of diabetes usually makes its unwelcome appearance in childhood, adolescence, or early adulthood. Only about 5 to 10 percent of Americans diagnosed with diabetes have type one. The more common form of the disease, type two diabetes, results from the body's inability to make enough insulin or to properly use the insulin that it makes, a condition known as insulin resistance. Some individuals with type two diabetes may be able to keep their blood sugar levels under control with diet and exercise alone, while others may need to take oral medications on a daily basis. In rare cases, management of type two diabetes may ultimately include insulin injections.

It is estimated that a third of all people suffering from type two diabetes aren't even aware that they have the disease. That's why it is so important to be tested on a regular basis. Starting at the age of forty-five, your doctor will probably want to measure glucose levels in your blood every three years or so, even if you don't have any diabetic symptoms. Certain individuals should be tested earlier in life, as well as more frequently. Anyone who experiences symptoms of the disease, including excessive thirst or hunger; frequent urination; fatigue; or recurrent, slow-to-heal infections should be tested immediately. Folks who are overweight, have high triglyceride levels, or a family history of the condition may be advised to have the appropriate blood tests performed annually. Women who develop diabetes during a pregnancy, a condition known as gestational diabetes, will want to keep a close eye on their blood sugar levels forever. Nearly a third of women with gestational diabetes go on to develop type two diabetes later in life.

Obesity is a significant risk factor for diabetes, and in the wake of the skyrocketing incidence of obesity in the U.S., the rise in diabetes is following suit. Weight loss plays a critical role in the management of both conditions. Studies show that losing a modest amount of weight (often just ten pounds), and engaging in regular exercise can reduce the risk of developing type two diabetes by nearly 60 percent. If you have been diagnosed with diabetes, you'll want to work hard to keep your weight down and your blood sugar levels within an acceptable range. Complications of chronically elevated blood sugar levels include vision problems and blindness, heart and kidney disease, and nerve damage. These medical problems make up just a small part of an extremely long list.

Diabetes can dramatically affect sexual function in men and women, often within the first ten years of developing the condition. During this time frame, more than half of diabetic men will begin to notice early warning signs of erectile dysfunction (ED). The likelihood that ED will occur in diabetic men increases progressively with age. Between the ages of twenty and twenty-nine, fewer than 10 percent of diabetic men will have ED, but by the age of seventy, some 95 percent will be affected. At the vibrant age of sixty, more than half of all diabetic men will have some degree of erectile dysfunction.

Although sexual dysfunction in male diabetics has long been a topic of intense research and funding, the same interest in women has only recently surfaced. Despite the fact that women are more likely to develop diabetes than men, the female sexual implications of having the disease weren't even considered until the semi-enlightened years of the seventies. As a result, the medical community lags slightly behind in its understanding of sexual complications arising from the disease as they pertain to women. What *is* known is that up to a third of diabetic women develop chronic vaginal dryness and irritation. They also tend to experience noticeable deficiencies in genital sensation. Within the first four to six years of being diagnosed with the condition, many women report diminished interest and desire for sexual activity, as well as a reduction in their enjoyment of sexual intercourse.

For diabetic men and women, maintaining control of blood sugar levels will help reduce the risk of sustaining nerve damage in the long run, and increase the chances of expressing and enjoying your sexuality throughout your life.

HIGH CHOLESTEROL LEVELS

Thanks largely to the American "eat, drink, and be sedentary" way of life, high cholesterol levels are becoming an increasingly common problem in the U.S. Although heredity undoubtedly plays a role in promoting high cholesterol levels, eating too many high-fat and cholesterol-laden foods—especially meat and dairy products—is largely to blame.

Although cholesterol has several important purposes in life, including the manufacture of sex hormones and vitamin D, you really don't need to add any extra to your diet. Mother Nature has already assigned your liver the task of producing all that your body needs. When you force-feed your body excessive amounts of cholesterol by eating too many junk foods, fatty meats, and whole dairy products, the excess cholesterol leaks into your bloodstream and begins to accumulate on the walls of your blood vessels. Eventually, the buildup can slow, or even block, the flow of blood to the heart. Blood carries life-giving oxygen to the heart muscle. If oxygen-rich blood isn't able to penetrate a blockage in the coronary arteries leading to the heart, the heart muscle begins to suffer injury, and even death, resulting in a heart attack.

A desirable blood cholesterol level in people without heart disease is less than 200 milligrams per deciliter (mg/dL) of blood. Borderline-high cholesterol is considered to be in the range of 200 to 239 mg/dL, and levels greater than 240 mg/dL are typically considered high. The "good" type of cholesterol, called high-density lipoprotein (HDL) doesn't accumulate in blood vessels. In fact, it seems to actually help remove the dangerous buildup from along artery walls. The higher your HDL level the better, because high HDL levels are associated with a lower risk of having a heart attack. On the other hand, a HDL of less than 35 mg/dL is considered to be too low.

Low-density lipoprotein (LDL), is the "bad" type of cholesterol that sticks to the artery walls and creates blockages. As such, it is one of the most important risk factors for heart disease. The higher your LDL levels the greater your risk; and the lower your LDL, the better. For people without heart disease, a desirable LDL level is one that falls below 130 mg/dL.

Having high cholesterol levels not only bumps up your risk of developing heart disease and suffering a heart attack, it also dramatically increases your chances of experiencing sexual arousal disorders or erectile dysfunction (ED). Although large-scale research in women is lacking, one study found that as many as 38 percent of women with sexual arousal disorders also had abnormal cholesterol profiles. In the majority of these women, the cholesterol abnormalities had not previously been detected, much less treated. The results of the study indicate that the higher a woman's cholesterol level, the greater degree of dysfunction she is likely to experience during sexual arousal.

Studies involving male patients show that high cholesterol levels can increase a man's risk of developing ED by a whopping 80 percent. High cholesterol levels leading to plaque buildup in the arteries of the penis are thought to be responsible for nearly 70 percent of ED cases in men aged sixty and older. The association between erectile dysfunction and elevated cholesterol levels is so strong that the American Heart Association now advises doctors to evaluate all of their patients with ED for the presence of heart disease.

If your cholesterol levels aren't exactly ideal, chances are great that at some point in your life, your heart and your sexual performance will begin to suffer. Regular exercise, weight loss, and a low-fat diet can go a long way toward improving your cholesterol profile, as well as the health of your heart and your sex life. If lifestyle measures prove to be insufficient, your doctor may recommend taking a cholesterol-lowering drug. Some of these drugs can have a negative impact on sexual function. If this is the case, you may have to try a few cholesterol-lowering medicines before you find one that improves your health without diminishing your sexuality.

HIGH BLOOD PRESSURE

High blood pressure, sometimes called hypertension, is a relatively common problem in the U.S., affecting nearly a quarter of American adults. Healthy blood pressure is typically considered to be in the neighborhood of 120/80. The top number of the fraction (systolic blood pressure) represents the arterial pressure in millimeters of mercury as the heart muscle contracts. The bottom number (diastolic blood pressure) represents the pressure as the heart relaxes between beats. For hypertensive patients who are being treated with blood-pressure-lowering medications, the goal of therapy is to lower the pressure to a point below 140/90, and many doctors now recommend keeping it even lower.

Effective management of high blood pressure is critical to overall health. Not only does it reduce the risk of suffering a heart attack or stroke, it may also help improve sexual function. High blood pressure and sexual dysfunction appear to go hand in hand in both men and women. Although few studies have examined the effects of hypertension on female sexuality, those performed in male populations reveal that at least two-thirds of men with high blood pressure also have some degree of ED. About 40 percent of all cases of ED in the U.S. are thought to be attributable to the combination of hypertension and high cholesterol levels.

Elevated blood pressure increases the workload of the heart, placing a significant strain on the muscle itself, as well as on blood vessels throughout the body. Over time, these vessels can grow narrow, and become stiffer and harder. As arteries become less elastic, they exert more pressure. and the harder the heart must work to overcome the resulting resistance. Given the fact that the blood vessels supplying the genitals in men and women are rather distant from the heart, it's not hard to see how having high blood pressure can interfere with proper blood flow to the area. Reduced blood flow to the genital area means a slower, weaker sexual response, creating problems with arousal in women and erection in men.

Although there is little doubt that high blood pressure spells trouble for sexual performance, men and women with hypertension and sexual dysfunction should consider another possibility. In reality, the hypertension itself may not be the only factor interfering with their sex lives; it could be a side effect of the medicine they're taking to treat the condition. Anti-hypertensive medications are grouped into eight main classes of drugs, according to their mechanism of action. To complicate matters, some pills combine two or more of these medications. The result is a confusing array of more than one hundred drugs, any one of which can potentially interfere with libido and sexual performance. On the other hand, with all these choices, surely you and your doctor can find at least one that will control your blood pressure without putting a damper on your sex life.

OBESITY

If you're overweight, you're in very good company. Obesity is a national epidemic, and America has the depressing distinction of being the fattest nation in the world. The National Institutes of Health estimates that more than 60 percent of Americans are currently overweight or obese, and this number is on the rise.

The bad news is that obesity isn't just a cosmetic problem. Each year, nearly 300,000 Americans will lose their lives to complications arising from this deadly disease. Nearly two-thirds of overweight adults have at least one weight-related medical problem that is putting their health, and even their lives, at risk. In addition to decreasing life expectancy, obesity significantly increases the risk for developing other serious medical conditions. Obesity-related illnesses include heart disease, high blood pressure, high cholesterol, diabetes, and depression. If this list sounds familiar to you, it should—it reads very similarly to the list of problems associated with low libido and sexual dysfunction.

You may reluctantly acknowledge that you're a little overweight, but you might not be sure what you should weigh for optimum health. The latest, greatest tool for determining your desirable body weight is called the Body Mass Index (BMI).

The BMI is a measurement that plots your weight against your height to determine whether you are of normal weight, overweight, or obese. It is generally considered to be a more reliable marker of obesity than the old height-weight tables, and has recently been promoted to gold-standard status as a tool for measuring obesity. More importantly, it is useful in determining whether or not your weight is putting your health at risk. While the BMI is a useful index of obesity, it isn't entirely foolproof. For starters, it doesn't take into account the muscle-to-fat ratio of your body. If you're a large, muscle-bound athlete, you could be classified as "obese" on the basis of BMI, when in fact your buff bod doesn't have an ounce of excess body fat. If, on the other hand, you haven't exercised a lick since the last phys ed class of your senior year in high school, you could have a body composed almost entirely of flab, and still end up with a normal BMI. In spite of these shortcomings, the BMI is usually sufficient to assess the weight status of most people.

The optimal BMI for good health is thought to be in the range of 19 to 21 for women and 20 to 22 for men. If your BMI is a little greater, don't panic. Anyone with a BMI of 18.5 to 24.9 is still considered to be of normal weight. If you find that you have a BMI of 25 to 29, you probably really are overweight, and it's time to get moving with that exercise program you've been thinking about.

In general, a BMI of 24 or lower is consistent with good health as it relates to weight, while a BMI of 27 or greater is associated with an increased risk of developing type two diabetes, heart disease, stroke, and some types of cancer— not to mention sexual dysfunction.

DETERMINING YOUR BODY MASS INDEX (BMI)

The table below has already done the math and metric conversions. To use the tble, find the approprite height in the left-hand column. Move across the row to the given weight. the number at the top of the column is the BMI for that height and weight.

BMI (KG/M²)	19	20	21	22	23	24	25	26	27	28	29	30	35	40
HEIGHT (IN.)	WEIGHT (LB.)													
58	91	96	100	105	110	115	119	124	129	134	138	143	167	191
59	94	99	104	109	114	119	124	128	133	138	143	148	173	198
60	97	102	107	112	118	123	128	133	138	143	148	153	179	204
61	100	106	111	116	122	127	132	137	143	148	153	158	185	211
62	104	109	115	120	126	131	136	142	147	153	158	164	191	218
63	107	113	118	124	130	135	141	146	152	158	163	169	197	225
64	110	116	122	128	134	140	145	151	157	163	169	174	204	232
65	114	120	126	132	138	144	150	156	162	168	174	180	210	240
66	118	124	130	136	142	148	155	161	167	173	179	186	216	247
67	121	127	134	140	146	153	159	166	172	178	185	191	223	255
68	125	131	138	144	151	158	164	171	177	184	190	197	230	262
69	128	135	142	149	155	162	169	176	182	189	196	203	236	270
70	132	139	146	153	160	167	174	181	188	195	202	207	243	278
71	136	143	150	157	165	172	179	186	193	200	208	215	250	286
72	140	146	154	162	169	177	184	191	199	206	213	221	258	294
73	144	151	159	166	174	182	189	197	204	212	219	227	265	302
74	148	155	163	171	179	186	194	202	210	218	225	233	272	311
75	152	160	168	176	184	192	200	208	216	224	232	240	279	319
76	156	164	172	180	189	197	205	213	221	230	238	246	287	328

Body Weight in pounds according to height and body mass index.

Obesity and Sexuality

Even in the absence of the other debilitating diseases that it tends to travel with, obesity can—in and of itself—reduce libido and impair sexual function. As your native fat cells grow larger and larger, they begin to act as a separate gland with its own agenda. This "fat gland" can easily become the largest, most domineering gland in the body and can have profound negative effects on the entire system.

Fat cells contain aromatase, an enzyme that specializes in converting testosterone to estrogen. As the "fat gland" increases in size, aromatase production increases. Overweight individuals, whether male or female, will progressively lose testosterone, while estrogen levels continue to climb. Numerous studies have linked obesity with lowered testosterone levels at all ages. For both men and women, suboptimal levels of testosterone can dampen libido and lead to less than spectacular sexual performance and enjoyment. In severe cases, it can result in sexual dysfunction.

Biological issues aside, obesity can interfere with sexuality in other ways. Numerous studies have shown that people who are obese suffer from poor body image, which often leads to a lack of sexual self-confidence. By itself, being overweight or obese doesn't doom you to the development of a poor body image. Plenty of overweight men and women enjoy a great deal of self-confidence. But the majority of overweight and obese people are unhappy with their appearance, and it is this dissatisfaction that can lead to a poor body image. The worse you feel about your weight, the greater the impact your obesity has on your body image, self-esteem, and sexual self-confidence.

Some overweight individuals fear that their partners will reject them sexually on the basis of weight. In reality, this doesn't seem to be the norm. In a study of obese people and their sexual partners, 75 percent of participants stated that weight was rarely or never an issue in their relationships. Nearly the same number believed that their partners were very sexually attracted to them. Of the overweight subjects, nearly 94 percent said that they had rarely or never been on the receiving end of verbal abuse from their partners, at least as far as their weight was concerned. Most of the overweight participants felt very secure in their relationships. More than 80 percent said that they did not believe that their partners would find them less desirable in the unfortunate event that they gained even more weight.

In spite of these findings, there remains a strong link between obesity and poor body image. Poor body image, in turn, is highly correlated with sexual avoidance. If your weight status is sapping your self-esteem and sexual self-confidence, it is critical that you do something about it. You don't have to achieve massive weight loss to get a dramatic boost to your self-image. A loss of just five or ten pounds may be all it takes, and exercise is undoubtedly the best way to get the ball rolling. A regular exercise program also provides you with a few bonus benefits. You'll feel better physically and emotionally, and have more energy and stamina. While you're taking positive measures to improve your health and happiness, your sex life will also reap the benefits.

THYROID DISEASE

In its role as the master gland, the thyroid's function has a profound impact on all other glands, and ultimately on the hormonal milieu of the body. When it isn't functioning properly, all systems may suffer. Because this gland interacts with all others, any problem with the thyroid may create a glitch in the production of the sex steroids, and consequently lead to sexual dysfunction.

Thyroid disease is only rarely responsible for sexual dysfunction, but it is always a possibility. Disorders of the thyroid gland should be considered in any complete medical work up for sexual dysfunction, especially those occurring in women. Although the inability to achieve sexual arousal or erection isn't a classic sign of thyroid disease, the fatigue that accompanies an underactive thyroid gland is occasionally to blame for a lackluster libido.

As it turns out, women are diagnosed with thyroid disease about ten times more often than are men. While most doctors agree that there isn't much you can do to prevent the disease, you can keep yourself as healthy as possible by learning to recognize its warning signs and symptoms, and have it treated as soon as possible. There is some evidence to suggest that thyroid disease can be an inherited condition, so be sure to tell your doctor if there's a history of it in your family.

Your doctor will probably want to check your thyroid for enlargement, as well as the presence of lumps and bumps by feeling it with his fingers. In almost every case in which suspicion of thyroid disease exists, blood tests will be ordered to determine the levels of your various thyroid hormones. If your levels are found to be low, you'll probably be given a diagnosis of hypothyroidism, which indicates an underactive gland. Symptoms associated with this condition include constipation, weight gain, and fatigue. Individuals with underactive thyroid glands often complain of feeling mentally dull or sluggish. They tend to feel chilly when others around them are comfortable, and may notice that they have dry skin, coarse hair, and a tendency to look and feel bloated or puffy.

Armed with a diagnosis of hypothyroidism, your doctor will undoubtedly provide you with a prescription for synthetic thyroid hormone pills, which are usually taken in very small doses once a day. Although there are natural varieties of thyroid hormone available, most doctors are more comfortable prescribing the synthetic ones, which seem to be more reliable in terms of providing standard doses and predictable outcomes. The good news is that taking the medication will undoubtedly make you feel and act like yourself again, restoring your energy levels and mental agility. The bad new is that it usually takes some time, patience, and additional blood work to get the dose of medication properly adjusted. In most cases, thyroid medications are well-tolerated and have very few side effects.

While thyroid gland malfunction often results in hypothyroidism, it can also trigger a condition called hyperthyroidism, in which the overactive gland produces an excess of thyroid hormones. Symptoms of hyperthyroidism include weight loss, nervousness, a rapid heart rate, sweating, trembling, and irritability. Blood tests are also used to diagnose hyperthyroidism, and once detected, you may face one of several treatment options. Taking an oral medication is occasionally sufficient to keep thyroid hormones in check, but sometimes your condition will warrant the use of radiation treatment or surgery to remove all or part of the thyroid gland. Fortunately, most cases of hyperthyroidism respond to treatment, and afterwards, you'll undoubtedly return to your former state of good health.

CANCER

In spite of the amazing and encouraging progress being made in the development of cancer treatment and cures, the diagnosis is still devastating and the disease is incredibly scary. Receiving a diagnosis of any type of cancer can intimidate the bravest of souls. Since survival and coping become top priorities for cancer survivors, sexuality often has to take a back seat.

If you've been diagnosed with cancer, you know that the treatments involved can sometimes seem every bit as bad as the disease itself. While you're weighing the risks and benefits of different medicines, treatments, and surgeries, be sure to ask your doctors about their potential effects on your sexuality, in both the short- and long-term. The more information you have, the more comfortable you'll be with your decisions. As you heal, it is very likely that your desire for intimacy and delight in making love will return. You'll want to make sure that the methods of cancer treatment that you choose allow you to enjoy these sensations as fully as possible.

SPINAL CORD INJURY

Because the nerves that control sexual response and genital sensation are often damaged in spinal cord injuries, it would seem logical to expect dire sexual consequences after any type of injury to the spinal cord itself. Fortunately, this isn't always the case. It's a common misconception that people who are paralyzed below the waist can't have sex, and furthermore, probably won't even want it. Research shows that among victims of spinal cord injuries, sexual desire remains intact, and many are able to experience very satisfying orgasms through sexual contact, and even fantasy.

Nearly two-thirds of women with spinal cord injuries report that they are satisfied with their sexual experiences. On the other hand, nearly the same percentage of women say that they are dissatisfied with the advice and counseling they received after their injuries or diagnoses. The lesson here is this: Don't let anyone tell you that you can't or won't continue to be sexually active after sustaining a spinal cord injury, even if paralysis is part of the picture.

In male patients, the most common form of sexual difficulty arising from an injury to the spinal cord is erectile dysfunction. Fortunately, this condition can be treated. Medications, including Viagra, have proven effective in many men who suffer ED after sustaining spinal cord injuries. Although no large-scale studies have been done to date, it is highly likely that the drug will help women to some degree as well.

CHRONIC FATIGUE SYNDROME

Not surprisingly, the condition known as chronic fatigue syndrome (CFS) emerged with the baby boomers, and may explain, at least in part, their notorious lack of libido. In the mid-eighties, CFS began striking the stressed-out workaholics in the prime of their fast-paced lives with a vengeance, suddenly rendering them incapable of doing it all. Once dubbed the "yuppie flu," CFS has a predilection for college-educated high-income earners, usually between the ages of twenty to forty. Although women are three times more likely to be diagnosed with the condition, men certainly aren't immune.

Chronic fatigue syndrome is characterized by debilitating fatigue—not just your typical, end-of-the day tiredness, but a pervasive, bone-deep type of weariness and weakness. It can make carrying out the most mundane activities of daily life seem nearly impossible.

After more than two decades of scientific research, doctors and scientists have yet to agree on the exact cause of CFS. Some believe it is predominantly a physical disorder, while others attribute it to psychological problems. Regardless of its cause, fatigue is often cited as a major factor in diminished libido. It can definitely interfere with the quality—and quantity—of sex. As most people with CFS will tell you, it's hard to make love when you're too tired to move.

If you are plagued by a pervasive sense of fatigue most of the time, it's important to search for the source of the problem. After a complete physical exam, your doctor likely will order blood tests to check your levels of glucose, iron, and thyroid hormones. Other tests may be performed to rule out infection, cancer, and heart disease. If no identifiable source for your fatigue is discovered, you'll probably be advised to make a few healthy changes in your diet and level of physical activity. Since stress is often at the root of the problem, your physician may recommend trying some stress-relieving tactics, or attending a stress management course. With a little patience and time, chronic fatigue usually resolves, with or without medical treatment.

AGING

Aging certainly isn't a disease. If you live long enough, it is an inevitable condition, and most people find it much preferable to the alternative. Among younger folks, including some doctors, the idea that sex might be important to mature men and women is often viewed with a dash of ridicule. In truth, sexual contact and intimacy remain important components of a fulfilling life, right up to the end.

Although sexuality remains of interest to older men and women, there are undoubtedly differences in the ways it is expressed with advancing age. After years of practice and hands-on experience, older adults have pretty much perfected their craft. Expressions of sexuality tend to evolve into something much more refined. Minus the distractions of clamoring children and career pressures, personal relationships tend to take on greater meaning and value. After years together, intimacy develops to such a degree that partners are often able to read the other's mind, and know exactly what he or she wants and needs. For older men and women, sex is an exhilarating affirmation of life and love, and an enchanting celebration of the past and present.

Considering that the average life span for American men is seventy-four years, and eighty years for women, some of the most exhilarating and fulfilling sexual encounters may still lie before you. With so much time ahead of you, you certainly don't want to call it quits when it comes to your sexuality. While studies show that the importance of maintaining sexual relationships declines with age, it doesn't fall off as much as you may think. For most older people, it remains a crucial element of a fulfilling life. In a survey conducted by the American Association of Retired Persons (AARP), nearly 60 percent of women reported that having a satisfying sexual relationship was one of the most important quality-of-life issues.

When it comes to gender differences among older Americans, men are more likely to place importance on sexual activity than women (59 percent versus 35 percent). The AARP study showed that roughly 61 percent of men and 50 percent of women felt that sexual activity is critical to a good relationship. When asked if they would be happy throwing in the towel and never having sex again; only 3 percent of men and 20 percent of women replied in the affirmative. So much for the notion that the interest in lovemaking gets lost in the process of aging.

Although most older Americans agree that having an active sex life throughout their golden years is important, not all of them are as active as they would like to be. This phenomenon is undoubtedly due to the increased incidence of sexual dysfunction in men and women as they age. Although aging is frequently associated with sexual dysfunction, it isn't necessarily a life-sentence of celibacy. Older men and women who take good care of their emotional and physical health can expect to enjoy the act of lovemaking for years to come.

If you've reached the status of an "older person," and if sex is important and enjoyable to you, congratulations! Keep up the good work! Don't let anyone try to shame you into giving up your sexuality, or tell you that it shouldn't be important, enjoyable, or even possible. If your doctor doesn't take your sex life as seriously as you do, it might be time to think about finding one who will.

DEPRESSION

In your journey through life, you'll undoubtedly experience feelings of sadness from time to time, and these feelings are normal in many cases. Feeling a little low or down in the dumps on occasion is to be expected, and it doesn't necessarily mean that you've earned yourself a diagnosis of depression. When doctors and other medical specialists use the term "depression," they're referring to its clinical meaning, namely, major depression. Individuals diagnosed with major depression have all or most of the symptoms listed below almost every day, throughout the day, for two weeks or longer. Minor depression, as its name implies, is a less serious form of depression with less debilitating symptoms. Since major and minor depression often share similar causes, treatment for either may involve the same medications and behavioral therapies.

Although the exact changes that occur with depression aren't fully understood, it is thought that the condition results from an imbalance of neurochemicals in the brain. When you don't have enough of the "feel good" types of neurochemicals, or when your brain doesn't respond to them normally, you may become depressed. It is known that depression can be hereditary, and it is commonly linked to stressful life events, including the death of a loved one, divorce, or loss of a job. It isn't uncommon for people who suffer from chronic illnesses, especially advanced heart disease or cancer, to suffer from depression.

At any given time in the U.S., more than seventeen million people are battling depression. Women are nearly twice as likely to develop the condition as are men. About 20 to 25 percent of women will experience depression at least once during their lifetime, compared to just seven to 12 percent of men. The gender gap first appears during adolescence; then peaks during the menopausal period.

In spite of common misconceptions to the contrary, depression isn't a sign of weakness, nor is it a personality flaw. People with the condition usually aren't able to just "shake it off" or "get over it," no matter how hard they might try. Fortunately, depression can be treated, just like diabetes or high blood pressure. If your doctor diagnoses you with depression, she'll probably offer you a prescription antidepressant medication, with the goal of correcting the chemical imbalances in your brain. You may not experience the maximum beneficial effect of the drug for a month or two, so it's important not to give up on your medication—or yourself—before it's had a chance to work. Most doctors recommend staying on an antidepressant medication for at least six months.

Symptoms of Depression

- Lack of interest or loss of pleasure in activities that you once enjoyed, including sex
- Feeling sad or numb
- Crying easily or for no apparent reason
- Feeling restless, irritable, or sluggish
- Change in appetite, with unintentional change in weight
- Trouble remembering things, concentrating, and making decisions
- Headaches, body aches, and digestive problems
- Trouble sleeping, or wanting to sleep all the time
- Fatigue
- Recurrent thoughts about death or suicide

Depression and Sexuality

Depression has a powerful impact on libido, and low libido, in turn, can sometimes lead to depression in both men and women. Individuals suffering from depression have a higher prevalence of disorders of desire and sexual function than the general population. Although the relationship between depression and diminished desire frequently overlaps, one thing is certain: treatment of one condition often leads to improvements in the other.

There is evidence to suggest that the decline in libido is directly related to the depth of depression: The greater the degree of depression, the lower the libido. One large study found that more than 70 percent of depressed patients experienced a loss of sexual interest, even when they were not taking any type of antidepressant medication. Those suffering from the condition reported that the loss of sexual interest was more disturbing to them than any other symptom of depression. While the libido-leaching effects of depression are bad enough, side effects of the medicines used to treat the condition can worsen the problem. It is estimated that over 40 percent of people taking antidepressant medications experience some type of sexual dysfunction. The drugs most commonly prescribed for the treatment of depression are notorious for their libido-zapping effects.

Fortunately, not all people taking antidepressants experience diminished libido. In some, the medications can lift the spirits to the degree that sexual desire is actually increased. Even among these individuals, the medications still may work to interfere with the physiological sexual response and the ability to achieve orgasm. This phenomenon can lead to performance anxiety, a serious problem for many individuals, since more than 60 percent of depressed patients have coexisting anxiety. With anxiety, the "fight or flight" reaction is often triggered, and this chain reaction of events in the body's nervous system can completely shut down any type of sexual response.

Depression can be brought on by the hormonal, physical, and neurological changes that accompany menopause and andropause. Substance abuse, including excessive intake of alcohol, may lead to depression, and is occasionally at the root of sexual dysfunction and disorders of desire. Several studies have shown that individuals suffering from depression are more likely to abuse drugs and alcohol than those in the general population.

When depression improves with treatment, but libido remains low, it becomes important to examine the side effects of medications. Several large studies examining the prevalence of sexual dysfunction among antidepressant users found that medications belonging to the drug class known as the selective serotonin reuptake inhibitors (SSRIs) were associated with high rates of sexual dysfunction. On the other hand, Wellbutrin (bupropion) and Serzone (nefazone), drugs that fall outside the SSRI class, were credited with causing significantly lower rates of sexual dysfunction. A study conducted at the University of Virginia showed that of the antidepressants commonly used, Wellbutrin was associated with the lowest rate of sexual dysfunction, producing problems in 22 percent of the study population. In contrast, the SSRI drugs, Prozac (fluoxetine), Paxil (paroxetine), Zoloft (sertraline), and Celexa (citralopram) caused sexual dysfunction in about 40 percent of the patients. Another drug included in the study was Effexor (venlafaxine), a medication that is a mixed serotonin and norepinephrine reuptake inhibitor. Effexor was also associated with sexual dysfunction in approximately 40 percent of the subjects. Fortunately, most doctors are aware of the libido-diminishing effects of depression and antidepressant medication, and are more than willing to work with you to improve your sexual state of affairs. Changing your medications or adjusting the dosage may make it possible to strike a happy balance.

CHAPTER 6

DESIRE AND THE FEMALE LIFE CYCLE

CHANGES RELATED TO THE MANY SEASONS OF A WOMAN'S REPRODUCTIVE LIFE can profoundly impact her libido. Many of the conditions that accompany these changes present unique challenges and potential obstacles to sexuality. For some women, medication or surgery will ultimately be required to correct the problems that arise. Fortunately, the majority of women can remedy the situation just by making a few positive lifestyle changes.

PREMENSTRUAL SYNDROME

Here's the good news about PMS: It's not all in your head.. For years, the monthly monster known as premenstrual syndrome, or PMS for those of us on a first name basis, was dismissed as an ugly figment of the female imagination. Although many doctors and scientists are just now catching on, PMS-sufferers and their partners have always known that the condition is real, and furthermore, that it interferes dramatically with libido and sexual function.

Now that the medical community has seen the light, PMS has achieved the status of a respectable medical disorder. Although the actual prevalence of the condition is still unknown, an estimated 75 percent of women report the predictable occurrence of PMS symptoms with their monthly periods. The other 25 percent of women are either inordinately blessed—or else living in total denial. Thirty to 40 percent of women have symptoms severe enough to disrupt their daily lives, and about 7 percent have a form of PMS so disabling that it has earned its own psychiatric designation, premenstrual dysphoric disorder, or PMDD for short.

If you suffer pre-menstrual miseries, you've probably learned to brace yourself for the onslaught of physical and emotional changes that strike the week before your period. Moods can turn on a dime, flip-flopping between overwhelming sadness, grouchiness, and rip-roaring rage. Fatigue, food cravings, and sleep disturbances aren't uncommon. Constipation, abdominal bloating, and ankle swelling can make you feel like the Pillsbury Doughgirl, while memory lapses and trouble concentrating can leave you feeling more like a premenstrual dodo. The exact cause of PMS remains a mystery, but most experts believe that chemical changes in the brain and fluctuating hormone levels are the main triggers. Low levels of vitamins and minerals may also play a role, but it's likely that all these factors contribute to the condition and its symptoms to some degree.

If you have PMS, you can help yourself by making a few simple lifestyle changes. Engaging in regular exercise and adopting a sensible, nutritious diet are the best places to start. Foods that are rich in complex carbohydrates, like whole grains, cereals, and vegetables help keep your moods on an even keel. Although you may find yourself craving foods made of simple carbohydrates, like potato chips, chocolate, and other sweets, complex carbohydrates are far better choices. They have nutrients that help boost levels of serotonin, a neurotransmitter that is known to promote a sense of well-being. It's also a good idea to hold the salt during the week before your period. This will help reduce fluid retention, bloating, and the likelihood that you'll overreact to the presence of any water weight gain. Alcohol should be off-limits during this time: It only serves to aggravate depression and fatigue. Since caffeine contributes to breast tenderness and anxiety, you might want to go easy on the coffee and colas for a week or so around the time of your period.

Some researchers believe that adding key vitamins and minerals to your diet can banish PMS. Many doctors recommend taking 400 international units (IU) of Vitamin E daily to help alleviate symptoms. Vitamin E may dampen the effects of prostaglandins, the hormone-like chemicals that are blamed for many PMS-related miseries, like irritability, breast tenderness, and bloating. Calcium has been shown to improve the symptoms of PMS. A 1998 study published in the *American Journal of Obstetrics and Gynecology* found that women who took twelve hundred milligrams of chewable calcium carbonate daily experienced a 50 percent reduction in most of their PMS symptoms by the third month of treatment. Another study found that taking 200 milligrams of magnesium every day reduced PMS symptoms by 40 percent.

If lifestyle changes and supplements don't ease your suffering, your doctor might be able to help. Relief often comes in the form of a pill—*the* Pill to be exact. Oral contraceptives help regulate menstrual cycles and reduce your body's state of hormonal upheaval. If you don't like the idea of taking hormones to control your hormones—or your PMS symptoms—antidepressant drugs belonging to the selective serotonin reuptake inhibitor (SSRI) class may be a better solution. These drugs have been shown to cut PMS symptoms in half in 60 to 70 percent of women who take them.

Although there are no surefire diagnostic tests for PMS, a litany of symptoms may be all that your physician requires to recognize the condition. Keeping a monthly diary of miseries will help your doctor make the correct diagnosis, and more importantly, prescribe the most effective treatments.

Premenstrual Dysphoric Disorder

In spite of its intimidating title, premenstrual dysphoric disorder can really be thought of as a more serious form of PMS. It is estimated that from 2 to 10 percent of reproductive-aged women have severe distress and dysfunction caused by PMDD. It's not really surprising that women have so many physical and emotional changes during their periods. Menstruation is a time of complete hormonal upheaval, and the hormones doing all of the up-heaving have major impact on the brain, as well as the body.

While women with mild to moderate PMS symptoms may benefit from lifestyle changes and nutritional supplements, those with PMDD may need a little extra assistance. Women with PMDD who fail to respond to conservative measures may also require medications, which typically begin with a SSRI antidepressant. Medications in this class of drugs have been shown to dramatically reduce emotional, behavioral, and physical symptoms, resulting in improvements in psychosocial functioning. Even if you think you can survive the symptoms of PMDD without relying on medications, you might want to consider taking them to preserve harmony in the relationships that are most important to you.

While SSRI antidepressants and birth control pills are the medicines most commonly prescribed to treat PMDD, both can interfere with libido and can lead to sexual dysfunction. Whether or not to take either type of drug ultimately boils down to a type of cost-benefit situation. If taking a pill dampens your desire but improves your mood, making it possible to at least speak civilly to your partner, you may still come out ahead. Undoubtedly, the best solution is one that results in a win-win situation.

Intermittent dosing of the SSRI medications may improve the likelihood of favorable results. SSRI antidepressants including Prozac (fluoxetine), Celexa (citalopram), and Zoloft (sertraline) have been shown to be most effective when used only at key points in the menstrual cycle. Many doctors recommend a regimen that consists of taking the medications just two weeks out of the month, starting on the fourteenth day of the menstrual cycle. This dosing schedule seems to be just as effective as daily dosing, and studies show that SSRI medications are typically more effective than the Pill in treating PMDD. By taking the antidepressant drugs on an intermittent basis, you'll reduce the cost of the medication, as well as the likelihood of experiencing any long-term side sexual side effects.

Although PMDD is often considered to be a severe form of PMS, psychiatrists are more inclined to view it as a kind of depressive disorder, emphasizing its emotional and behavioral components. They may be onto something, because as it turns out, features of PMDD and depressive disorders overlap considerably. Symptoms of "atypical depression," including depressed moods, interpersonal rejection hypersensitivity (you think everybody hates you), carbohydrate cravings, and excessive sleeping are also characteristic of PMDD. Between one and two-thirds of women diagnosed with PMDD have a lifetime history of depression, compared to 15 percent of women without PMDD. Your doctor can help determine if your symptoms are related to PMDD or depression, and together you can decide on the appropriate treatment.

Treatment Approaches to PMDD
Lifestyle changes
- Eat small, frequent meals that are rich in complex carbohydrates and low in simple sugars, salt, fat, and caffeine.
- Get regular exercise.
- Get at least thirty minutes of sunshine every day. (Don't forget to wear your sunscreen!)
- Nix the cancer sticks—stop smoking.
- Go easy on the alcohol.
- Get plenty of sleep, and stick to a regular schedule if possible.

Nutritional Supplements
- Vitamin B6, 100 mg per day
- Vitamin E 400 IU per day
- Calcium Carbonate 1200 to 1500 mg per day
- Magnesium, 200 mg per day
- Tryptophan, 6 mg per day

Counseling
- Stress and anger management
- Assertiveness training
- Support groups (a couple of girlfriends and a night out can work wonders)

CONTRACEPTION: BIRTH CONTROL PILLS

When drug companies introduced their updated versions of the Pill in the mid-eighties, they claimed that their new and improved models were less likely to cause unwelcome side effects. What they didn't know was that the newer "triphasic" pills hold an even greater advantage over their predecessors: they may enhance a woman's sex drive. While peering into the erotic activities of Pill users, researchers at San Francisco State University took it upon themselves to ask their collegiate volunteers which kind of birth control pills they were currently taking. About three women in five were using the older monophasic varieties, the types that provide users with a constant level of synthetic hormones. The remaining women in the study were taking the newer triphasic types, in which the dosage changes every week or so, the better to mimic the biological and hormonal profile of a woman's menstrual cycle.

Although both kinds of pills are effective in doing what they're designed to do—prevent pregnancy—the researchers found that co-eds who were taking the triphasic tablets seemed to be having more fun in their extracurricular excursions, including sexual activities. Women taking the triphasic pills even reported thinking and fantasizing about sex more often than those taking the older varieties of the Pill. The triphasic-taking women also enjoyed a greater degree of sexual arousal and lubrication during lovemaking.

In light of these findings, the researchers speculated that the monophasic varieties of birth control pills tend to suppress a woman's natural hormones, which serve meaningful roles as aphrodisiacs. In contrast, by fluctuating throughout a woman's menstrual cycle, the triphasic varieties of the Pill tend to have less censorship over a woman's own romance-seeking hormones. Because women taking the triphasic pills haven't yet been compared to those not using any form of oral contraceptive, it isn't known whether or not the triphasic users have any type of sexual advantage over those women who remain Pill-less.

Oral contraceptives can impair libido and sexuality to such an extent that nearly a third of all Pill users stop taking it after just three months. Because the Pill suppresses the activity of the ovaries, it undoubtedly lowers testosterone production. This effect is intensified by the Pill's tendency to increase levels of a substance known as sex hormone binding globulin (SHBG) in the blood. As its name implies, SHBG binds to sex hormones in the body, reducing their bioavailability, and thus their ability to influence cells and tissues throughout the body. As the Pill drives up SHBG levels, more of a woman's libido-enhancing testosterone is rendered inactive, and less is available to work its magic in the sexual desire department.

In spite of being a relatively common problem, the issue of the libido-squashing side effects of the Pill have been basically ignored for most of the forty years that oral contraceptives have been in use. It is interesting to note that as scientists at major pharmaceutical companies race to develop an effective oral contraceptive for men, the issue of libido is of *paramount* importance. So much for equality.

PREGNANCY

Pregnancy and the postpartum period are often associated with a bewildering array of emotional, physical, and hormonal changes. Decreases in sexual desire, activity, and satisfaction are not uncommon during these periods, and they can linger on throughout the lactation period. Hopefully, they'll end well before the little bundle of joy reaches his first birthday, or at least by the time he graduates from college.

Myths, wives tales, and horror stories about the dangers of having sex during pregnancy abound. The truth is, having sexual intercourse is generally safe for most women with healthy pregnancies. On the other hand, if your doctor tells you that you're at risk for experiencing premature labor, or that you have a weakened or "incompetent" cervix, that's a whole different story.

Absent any complications or special risk factors, most expectant women can enjoy—or at least try to enjoy—lovemaking well into the third trimester. If lovemaking causes bleeding, pain, or contractions, you should stop, and talk to your doctor before you try again.

Many expectant couples are concerned that intercourse will cause a miscarriage, especially in the first trimester of pregnancy. In almost all cases, miscarriages are unrelated to sexual activity. More common causes are genetic defects in the developing fetus, hormonal insufficiencies in the mother, and some types of infection. If all is well with your pregnancy, having intercourse won't harm your baby. During sex, the penis doesn't come into actual contact with the fetus, which is well-protected by the amniotic fluid and the muscular layers of the womb. The mucous plug in the cervical canal prevents bacteria and semen from entering the womb, and this plug typically remains in place until delivery is imminent. In addition, you've undoubtedly got at least a small layer of abdominal and pelvic fat, and this serves to protect your developing baby from any external pressure applied by your partner.

Having an orgasm may cause the uterus to contract, even when you're not pregnant. The vast majority of studies indicate that in normal pregnancies, orgasms, with or without intercourse, don't lead to premature labor or premature birth. If at any point in your pregnancy, you develop vaginal bleeding, an incompetent cervix, preterm labor, or placenta previa (a placenta that covers the cervical opening), your doctor will likely invite you to stop having vaginal intercourse. If you're expecting twins or triplets, you may be advised to abstain from engaging in vaginal intercourse during the late second and early third trimesters, when preterm labor is most likely to occur. Even in normal pregnancies, your doctor may recommend total abstinence during the last few weeks of pregnancy as a precaution against triggering contractions that result in labor.

Decreased libido early in your pregnancy may play a significant role in your sexual activity. Rambunctious hormones, nausea, weight gain, and a profound sense of fatigue may totally wipe out your energy stores, as well as your sexual desire. Although your libido may take a downward plunge during the first trimester, you may find that your level of interest flares during the second trimester of pregnancy. Copious blood flow to your breasts and pelvis, compliments of the pregnancy, can take your interest and enjoyment in sex to a whole new level.

As you limp toward the finish line in your final trimester, you may find that your sexual desire takes a downward turn again. Having a pumpkin-sized belly can make intercourse physically challenging, to say the least. Given the limitations that your abdomen places on making love in more traditional positions, you and your partner can have fun experimenting with new ones that are more comfortable for both of you.

Although the level of sexual interest and physical abilities of the mother-to-be are often the limiting factors in the pregnant-sex equation, it's not always the case. It's not at all unusual for dads-to-be to feel a little tentative about making love to their pregnant wives. Fear of triggering a miscarriage or hurting the baby are contributing factors. Reassurance is helpful, and communication between partners becomes more important than ever.

As you enter the postpartum period immediately following the blessed event, your physical readiness for sexual intercourse will vary depending upon the circumstances of your delivery. In general, women who experience uncomplicated vaginal deliveries can resume sexual intercourse within three to six weeks, as long as both you and your partner are comfortable and there are no complicating factors. If you have questions, concerns, or doubts about the safety of resuming sexual activity, be sure to ask your doctor.

PERIMENOPAUSE

No matter how prepared you think you are, the transitional stage of life called "perimenopause" can still sneak up on you—and just when you were starting to get a handle on PMS. If you're smack dab in the middle of perimenopause, you aren't alone. Currently, over forty million women are in the same boat. Most women can expect to hit this hormonal hurricane head on around the age of forty-seven. They can look forward to spending an average of four to five years trapped in the transition zone before they officially cross the threshold into menopause.

While the average American woman experiences menopause at the age of fifty-one, about 8 percent of women become menopausal before the age of forty. If you're one of these early birds, perimenopausal symptoms could catch you totally off guard at the tender age of thirty-something. When this occurs as a result of natural causes, it is called "premature menopause." When it occurs as the result of a surgery or as a side effect of medication, it is called "surgical menopause."

No matter how old you are when perimenopause comes calling, the changes that accompany it can drive you to distraction. Although about 10 percent of women are lucky enough to go through this transitional period unscathed, most will experience a bewildering constellation of symptoms. Common complaints include hot flashes, night sweats, memory loss, insomnia, and irritability. Experiencing a nosedive in your level of libido and being introduced to the challenges posed by lack of bladder control can make matters worse.

Plummeting estrogen levels are to blame for most of these maladies, and as levels of the hormone continue to dwindle, you'll likely notice a change in your menstrual cycle. Even if you were once as regular as clockwork, you'll probably begin to skip a period here and there. Nearly 70 percent of women in their forties experience irregular menstrual bleeding, making it the most common—and inconvenient—symptom of perimenopause. Because they're skipping periods, many perimenopausal women are under the erroneous impression that they can't get pregnant. Some of these women will be in for a seven-pound surprise. Second only to teenagers, women in their forties have the next highest rate of unplanned pregnancies. If you're not planning to decorate the nursery, it's probably a good idea to keep using contraception throughout the perimenopausal period. Just to be on the safe side, you might want to consider continuing it for an entire year after your last menstrual period.

How do you know for sure that you're trapped in the throes of perimenopause? Unfortunately, there isn't any single test that can confirm the diagnosis. Your doctor may listen to your symptoms, and then make a judgment call. In making the diagnosis, physicians typically consider several factors, including your age, symptoms, and the results of blood tests that measure your hormone levels. Once you're given the dastardly diagnosis, you and your doctor can decide on the best way to treat it, if at all.

Since perimenopause really isn't an illness or a disease, you might be tempted to tough it out alone. If your symptoms are bringing you down, on the other hand, there's no need to be a perimenopausal martyr. A few prescription medications and natural remedies can help ease the transition.

Your doctor may advise you to take low-dose birth control pills. The Pill is usually the treatment of choice for women under fifty who don't smoke or have a history of breast cancer. Birth control pills work by shutting down your body's own erratic estrogen production and replacing it with a steady supply. Since fluctuating hormone levels are responsible for the majority of perimenopausal miseries, taking the Pill can completely eliminate symptoms like hot flashes, irritability, and insomnia. More importantly, oral contraceptives can regulate your menstrual periods and prevent pregnancy. Technically, the Pill could interfere with your libido. But for women whose hot flashes and other symptoms make having sex out of the question, taking the Pill might actually bring an end to a perimenopausally-induced sexual drought.

Even the lowest dose oral contraceptives contain several times the amount of estrogen used in traditional hormone replacement therapies. Since high doses of estrogen can increase breast cancer risk, it's a good idea to stop taking the Pill and switch over to conventional hormone replacement therapy when you graduate to menopause. If you aren't crazy about the idea of taking the Pill, you can always opt for the natural approach. Pharmacies and health food stores offer dozens of herbs and supplements that can soothe the symptoms of perimenopause and smooth the transition to menopause.

No matter how unwelcome the first signs of perimenopause may be, they can serve as an excellent wake-up call. If you've been thinking about making some positive, much-needed changes in your diet and exercise habits, there's no better time than now. It also provides the perfect excuse to see your doctor for a complete check-up.

HYSTERECTOMY

Hysterectomies are the second most common type of surgery performed in the U.S., taking a back seat only to Cesarean sections. Each year, nearly six hundred thousand women undergo the procedure. There's a great deal of controversy about whether either of the surgeries is absolutely necessary, or even in the best interest of the women who undergo them, but that's not the real issue here.

There are several types of hysterectomies, which vary in the degree to which the doctor removes pieces and parts of the patient's reproductive organs. All hysterectomies involve the removal of the uterus, or womb. A "total," or "complete hysterectomy," is a procedure in which the uterus and cervix are removed, while the ovaries are left in place. After undergoing this procedure, a woman will no longer get her menstrual periods, nor will she be able to bear children. Women in their reproductive years, however, will continue to ovulate, and their ovaries will still be capable of producing the hormones that so profoundly affect their health and sexuality.

When a woman undergoes a hysterectomy that involves the removal of all of her reproductive organs, the hormonal outcomes are quite different. This type of surgery, called a "total hysterectomy with bilateral salpingo-oophorectomy," is the most extensive type of hysterectomy, not to mention the hardest to pronounce. Following this procedure, a woman will no longer be capable of bearing children. Minus her ovaries, a woman of reproductive age will experience dramatic reductions in her levels of testosterone and estrogen, two hormones normally produced by the ovaries prior to menopause. As a result, she will plunge almost instantaneously into menopause, which in this case, is called "surgical" menopause.

MENOPAUSE

Menopause is defined as the absence of menstruation for one year. This definition is a source of frustration to many women, as the diagnosis can only be made in retrospect. Fortunately, most women are sufficiently in tune with their bodies that they don't need much help making the diagnosis. If you're around the age of fifty, you've ceased menstruating, and you're experiencing hot flashes, the diagnosis of menopause is a shoo-in. Still, if you have any questions about it, your doctor can help make the call. She may want to order blood tests to determine the levels of several hormones, including follicle-stimulating hormone (FSH) and estrogen. During menopause, FSH levels typically rise, while estrogen levels plummet. Depending on the outcomes of your tests, your doctor will determine whether or not you have crossed the threshold into the wonderful world of menopause.

These days, most women can expect to live to the ripe old age of eighty-plus. If you become menopausal around the age of fifty, you can look forward to spending about a third of your life in a postmenopausal state. Although it may not sound very inviting, it is infinitely better than the alternative. With so much time ahead of you, you'll want to make the most of your health and your sexuality. For most women, the two symptoms of menopause that produce the most misery are hot flashes and vaginal dryness, both of which tend to interfere with sexual desire. A few fortunate women will breeze through menopause without so much as breaking a sweat, but at least half of all menopausal women experience hot flashes for a grand total of five years.

While about 15 percent of menopausal women will sidestep hot flashes, vaginal dryness is practically inevitable. As women journey through menopause and beyond, vaginal dryness increases. Minus the nurturing effects of estrogen, the vaginal tissues tend to shrink and dry out, and produce fewer natural secretions. As if that weren't bad enough, the breasts and genitals become less sensitive, and orgasm less intense. Needless to say, all of these changes can make enjoying an active and fulfilling sex life a little challenging.

WHAT'S HAPPENING TO MY BODY? CHANGES AT MENOPAUSE

- *Skin:* Decreased activity of sweat and sebaceous glands, decreased sensation

- *Breasts:* Decreased fat content of breasts, diminished breast swelling and nipple erectile response with sexual arousal

- *Vagina:* Shortening and loss of elasticity of the vaginal canal, diminished secretions, thinning of the mucous membranes

- *Internal reproductive organs:* Ovaries and uterus shrink, cervix degenerates and decreases mucous production

- *Urinary tract:* Urethra and bladder muscles shrink and weaken

Treatment for Menopause

Until recently, the quick and easy solution for easing menopausal symptoms came in the form of a prescription for hormone replacement therapy, usually consisting of estrogen and progestin. Of all the menopausal remedies, estrogen has consistently proven itself to be the most effective in symptom relief. As a result, estrogen/progestin replacement therapy has long been one of the most commonly used medical regimens in the U.S., taken by an estimated 38 percent of postmenopausal women in 2000.

That percentage took a hard nosedive in 2002, after data from the now famous Women's Health Initiative (WHI) study were released. Women taking estrogen plus progestin were found to have an increased risk of developing breast cancer within just three years of starting the regimen. The WHI study soundly disproved the theory that hormone replacement therapy reduced a woman's risk for heart disease. In fact, supplemental estrogen plus progestin was shown to boost the risk of cardiovascular disease in postmenopausal women. So compelling were the data supporting the negative effects of hormone replacement therapy that the women in the WHI study were taken off the hormone medication prematurely. Researchers felt it would be unethical to allow women to continue to take supplemental estrogen in the face of such damning evidence. Based on the WHI findings, estrogen/progestin therapy is now *cautiously* recommended for the short-term relief of menopausal symptoms, and most doctors advise women to limit its use to three years or less. Fortunately, there are natural and prescription alternatives to synthetic hormones. Some are effective in alleviating hot flashes and vaginal dryness, while others are known to enhance sexual desire.

Testosterone Supplements and Libido

In addition to the myriad physical changes that accompany menopause, many women experience a significant drop in libido. Although some of this drop is undoubtedly due to physical factors, it is known that hormonal changes associated with menopause dramatically influence sexual desire, even in the absence of physical changes.

In the five years preceding menopause, estrogen and testosterone levels in women begin to fall. During menopause, women typically experience an 80 percent drop in their estrogen levels, and a 50 percent reduction in testosterone levels. Both hormones have profound influences on sexual desire, and their reduction is probably responsible for the fact that after the age of fifty-five, women report nearly a 50 percent drop in sexual activity. This is unfortunate for several reasons. Research has shown that women who remain sexually active during menopause experience fewer negative physical changes associated with the change of life. At least one study supports the old "use it or lose it" theory: The more frequently women engage in sexual intercourse, the more likely they are to continue to desire it and enjoy it.

For menopausal women whose loss of libido is caused by dwindling testosterone levels, supplemental testosterone can work wonders. When you think of testosterone, you probably associate it with manly men with deep voices, bulging biceps, and hairy chests. It's true that testosterone is the essence of masculinity, but it's also a woman's hormone. In the years between puberty and menopause, testosterone is manufactured and secreted by the female ovaries and adrenal glands, although much of it is ultimately converted into the female hormone estrogen. The total amount of free testosterone circulating in a woman's body is miniscule: roughly twenty times less than that of an adult male. Nonetheless, it is an essential amount, and receptors for testosterone can be found in many tissues throughout the female body, including the brain and sex organs.

Although the adrenal glands normally continue to manufacture small amounts of estrogen and testosterone after menopause, the ovaries stop making it altogether, and testosterone levels fall rather dramatically. Women who take estrogen replacement therapy during menopause usually experience a welcome reduction in their menopausal symptoms, but the regimen may actually suppress libido even further. Taking supplemental estrogen drives up levels of sex hormone binding globulin (SHBG), which may in turn bind to free testosterone, making it less biologically available to fuel sexual desire.

While the effects of estrogen deficiency that occur with menopause are well-understood, far less is known about the full impact of low testosterone levels in postmenopausal women. Low testosterone levels, are, however, consistently associated with low libido. A recent study published in *JAMA* found that women with low testosterone levels are significantly more prone to fatigue, depression, and loss of libido than are women with higher levels.

Although doctors have been prescribing testosterone replacement therapy for men since the 1930s, it wasn't until recently that the treatment was considered acceptable for women. In spite of its many proven benefits, the treatment is still quite controversial. The potential for unwelcome side effects keeps many women from trying it, and many physicians from recommending it.

In a very small percentage of women, the use of supplemental testosterone may lead to a masculine deepening of the voice, the development of facial hair and male-pattern baldness, and the onset of acne. These side effects seldom occur at the low testosterone doses most often prescribed by doctors today, especially when administered simultaneously with estrogen. When they do occur, the changes are usually quickly reversed with a reduction in dosage.

Another potential consequence of supplemental testosterone is the unfavorable alteration of a woman's cholesterol profile. This hormone is known to slightly lower the concentration of high-density lipoprotein (HDL), or good cholesterol, in the bloodstream. Traditional estrogen replacement therapy, on the other hand, is generally associated with an improvement in HDL levels.

On the plus side, the addition of testosterone to traditional hormone replacement therapy has been shown to improve energy levels, enhance feelings of well-being, and dramatically bolster libido. For menopausal women who continue to experience hot flashes and night sweats even after taking estrogen, supplemental testosterone often provides relief. It also helps boost lean muscle mass, enhance short-term memory, and increase the elasticity of the skin, resulting in a younger-looking complexion.

Another benefit of testosterone replacement therapy in women is its ability to increase bone mass. Osteoporosis currently affects more than twenty eight million women in the U.S., and approximately 75 percent of these women are postmenopausal. While traditional estrogen replacement therapy is known to prevent the additional loss of bone, treatment with a combination of estrogen and testosterone goes one step further. Not only does it stop bone loss; it also helps strengthen the skeleton by stimulating the formation of new bone.

Supplemental testosterone in women has been shown to boost the motivational aspects of sexual behavior, increasing energy levels, libido, and sexual fantasy. It has also been shown to increase blood flow to the vagina, enhance sensitivity of the breasts and genitalia, and facilitate sexual arousal. Women taking supplemental testosterone are more likely to engage in sexual activity, and tend to derive greater satisfaction from it.

When it comes to taking supplemental testosterone, women's choices are limited by the availability of approved medications. Hormone replacement therapy consisting of estrogen and small amounts of testosterone is available in the form of a pill, and currently, the only FDA-approved estrogen-testosterone combination pill is Estratest. This drug contains what most experts believe to be a balanced combination of the two hormones.

While doctors commonly prescribe Estratest to treat low libido in menopausal women, it's use for this purpose is considered to be "off-label," meaning that the drug doesn't have the U.S. Food and Drug Administration's approval for the specific treatment of low libido. Estratest is approved only for the treatment of menopausal symptoms like hot flashes and night sweats. Nonetheless, numerous studies have found it highly effective for bolstering the female libido. Women considered to be the best candidates for combination estrogen-testosterone therapy are those who are currently taking traditional estrogen replacement therapy and continue to experience hot flashes or loss of libido, as well as women with an elevated risk for osteoporosis.

For women who can't or don't want to take combination estrogen-testosterone therapies, testosterone injections may provide a solution. Injections are typically given every two to four weeks, and most women find them very effective in enhancing sexual desire. Although currently there are no testosterone-containing prescription products that are FDA-approved for the specific purpose of treating low libido in women, many pharmacists are now formulating low-dose testosterone creams, gels, and lozenges for their patrons. Testosterone-containing creams and gels are typically applied several times a week to an area of the body where the skin is thin, to allow for easy absorption, and they are generally well tolerated and very effective. Testosterone-containing lozenges may be taken on a regular basis, or they may be used immediately prior to sexual activity. Testosterone creams, gels, and lozenges still require a doctor's prescription, as well as the services of a pharmacist who is skilled in compounding the products.

While studies have shown that testosterone patches are extremely effective in heightening women's sexual desire, they have yet to be approved for use in women by the FDA and are currently considered to be experimental. In a study of women who had been rendered menopausal after having their ovaries removed, those receiving twice-weekly testosterone patches in addition to oral estrogen replacement therapy showed significant improvements in sexual functioning and feelings of well-being. The percentage of women who engaged in sexual intercourse at least once a week nearly doubled among those using the patch. No significant side effects were associated with the use of the testosterone patch: Women using the therapy experienced no change in total cholesterol levels, unwanted body hair, or acne.

Based on the findings of this study, it is reasonable to conclude that testosterone replacement therapy, at least as provided by the testosterone patch, produces significant increases in libido, sexual functioning, and overall sense of well-being in women who have undergone surgical menopause. It is thought that these benefits also extend to women who have experienced menopause naturally. Although the skin patches aren't yet approved for use in women in the United States, it's likely that they will be in the near future.

Before prescribing supplemental testosterone to their female patients, many doctors order a battery of tests, including a Pap smear and a mammogram. Blood work is performed to determine a woman's hormonal status and to reveal any abnormalities in her liver function or cholesterol profile. A bone mineral density test is often used to evaluate the skeleton for signs of bone loss or osteoporosis. As long as a woman continues to use testosterone replacement therapy, her doctor will undoubtedly want to continue monitoring her health with regular blood tests and physical exams.

The goal of testosterone replacement therapy for women is not to transform them into masculine creatures with bulging biceps and hairy chests, but rather to replicate their pre-menopausal testosterone levels. For some women, a touch of testosterone may be all it takes to dramatically improve the quality of life.

As you explore hormone-based therapies, here's something to keep in mind: Given the biological, physical, and emotional differences among individuals, there's no single "right" way to go about hormone replacement therapy. The key to success if finding what works best for you and your body. You may have to give several different regimens a try before you and your doctor hit upon just the right mix for you. Even if your doctor has had amazing success with a certain hormonal regimen in several patients, you are perfectly within your rights to be different. If you don't respond to the therapy as expected or desired, don't be afraid to ask your doctor to continue to work with you until you do.

URINARY INCONTINENCE

A few things haven't changed since kindergarten, including the rules regarding potty breaks. If you've ever lost control of your bladder as an adult, you may have felt just as embarrassed as you did as a preschooler.

Although it may be embarrassing, involuntary loss of urine is not uncommon. Women are much more likely to be afflicted than men, for several reasons, including childbirth and menopause. Carting around those eight-pound babies in our bellies for nine months and then muscling them out during labor and delivery can weaken or injure our pelvic muscles and nerves.

Most of the muscles in the female pelvis depend on the hormone estrogen to keep them firm and strong. After menopause, the lack of estrogen renders these muscles loose and weak. The uterus and bladder may drop, causing urinary incontinence. Unlike hot flashes, leakage of urine doesn't go away—it tends to worsen over time. Loss of bladder control is one of the major reasons that elderly women are placed in nursing homes, which is rather ironic, considering the thousands of diapers the average woman changes in her lifetime.

Urinary incontinence isn't just a problem for elderly women. About one in every ten women under age sixty-five is affected, and of the women who suffer from urinary incontinence, about a third develop it before the age of thirty-five. Many affected women consider themselves to be at the peak of their sexuality. Unfortunately, the unexpected loss of urine often prevents them from enjoying sexual activity. In some women, the potential for embarrassment may cause them to avoid sex altogether.

There are several types of urinary incontinence, each with different causes, symptoms, and treatments. "Stress incontinence" is the involuntary loss of urine during sneezing, laughing, or in other situations that increase intra-abdominal pressure. A number of factors contribute to stress incontinence. Cardiovascular disease and diabetes are often at the root of the problem. Medications prescribed for unrelated conditions, such as diuretics for the treatment of hypertension, may be responsible.

This type is common immediately after childbirth, when the pelvic muscles are still recovering from the trauma of delivery. Stress incontinence is also relatively common in postmenopausal women.

Even in younger women, an overactive bladder can be problematic. In women under age fifty-five, bladder disorders are the second leading medical cause of loss of employment. Embarrassment and continuous discomfort can lead to isolation from others, including sexual partners. In spite of the magnitude of the problem, most women with overactive bladder don't seek or get the help they need.

"Urge incontinence" is the uncontrolled loss of urine immediately after experiencing a strong, unexpected urge to void. Hearing or touching running water, or even the simple act of drinking may be all that's needed to bring on the urge to urinate.

"Overflow incontinence" is more often diagnosed in women whose bladders have dropped because of weak pelvic muscles, but it's also typical in people with diabetes. This type of incontinence occurs when the bladder stays perpetually full. When an additional amount of urine is delivered to the bladder, it overflows, causing urine to dribble out of the afflicted person's body and onto her clothes.

If you have urinary incontinence, you may be a little embarrassed, but don't let it keep you from seeking help. Some types are reversible, and your doctor can help you launch an investigation for potential causes. Side effects of medications and infection are reversible causes. Even if your incontinence isn't easily cured, you're not doomed to a lifetime of dampness; there are more treatments available now than ever before.

Surgery can return a dropped bladder to its proper position, enlarge a small bladder, or support weakened pelvic muscles. But not everyone needs surgery—more conservative approaches to urinary incontinence can be effective.

A cure might be as simple as taking a single pill a day. Two medications commonly used in the treatment of incontinence are Detrol and Ditropan. These drugs are generally well tolerated, and they're often very effective. In addition to medications, behavioral modification techniques can help you gain control over some types of incontinence. They may just help you get back your life—and your sexuality.

Treatment for Urinary Incontinence

There are a few steps that you can take on your own to improve your bladder control. Avoid foods that are known to be irritating to the bladder, including citrus fruit and juices, tomatoes, and spicy foods. Try to limit your consumption of alcohol and caffeine-containing beverages, as both can trigger the urge to urinate. Whatever you do, don't stop drinking water. Drink at least five to six glasses of water a day—just avoid downing them within two hours of bedtime.

Since being overweight can sometimes contribute to bladder control problems, you might want to get started on that exercise program you've been postponing. While you're up and moving, throw out all your tight pants, girdles, and high heels. All of these torture devices make bladder control more difficult. If your bladder is misbehaving, you should definitely stop smoking. Chronic coughing caused by cigarette smoking can weaken the pelvic muscles, and the nicotine in the cigarettes can cause bladder contractions.

If you're willing to work a little, you can actually retrain your bladder muscles to hold urine for longer and longer periods. Try to urinate at frequent, regular intervals, starting with once every hour, and then progressively lengthening the interval. This practice, known as "bladder training," cures about 10 to 15 percent of women with urinary incontinence and significantly helps about 75 percent more. Doing pelvic muscle exercises, or Kegels, is an easy, effective way to strengthen the muscles that support your bladder. If you stick with them, you'll undoubtedly notice a big difference in bladder control. Kegels are easy to do: Just squeeze the muscles that you use when you stop your flow of urine, and then relax. Squeeze! Now relax for about ten seconds. And again! Relax. Try doing ten or fifteen repetitions two or three times each day. You may be amazed at the results. Kegel exercises improve bladder control in about 80 percent of otherwise healthy women.

For some folks, even Kegels don't improve bladder control. Not to worry: Doctors have a few more tricks up their sleeves. Recently, several new devices have been designed to help prevent loss of bladder control. One such device, marketed as Introl, is a soft, U-shaped insertible device that holds the bladder in the proper position. In clinical trials it kept about 80 percent of women dry. Another insertible device, dubbed Reliance, is a tiny disposable rubber balloon that can remain in place up to six hours, and can be removed whenever you want to urinate. If you suffer from urinary incontinence, see your doctor. In most healthy people, it's a problem that can be successfully treated.

CHAPTER 7

FROM ANDROPAUSE TO VASECTOMY:

Special Concerns for Men

WE'VE LOOKED AT HOW HEALTH CONDITIONS THAT AFFLICT BOTH MEN AND WOMEN affect sexual desire, and in some cases, performance. This chapter discusses that subset of health problems which are not only specific to men, but also affect the male reproductive system, and ultimately, male sexuality.

BENIGN PROSTATIC HYPERPLASIA

There's a reason why guys get grumpier with age—most have an annoying condition called "benign prostatic hyperplasia." The disorder, commonly known as BPH, is the non-cancerous growth of the prostate gland that occurs almost universally in aging men. Between the ages of forty and sixty-four, up to 20 percent of men will develop BPH, and more than 40 percent of men older than sixty will be afflicted. For men fortunate enough to make it to the grand old age of eighty, 90 percent will be affected by prostatic enlargement.

Besides making many men miserable in their golden years, the prostate gland's other purpose in life is to provide a fluid contribution to semen. Most men won't give their glands much thought until they reach the age of fifty or so. Prior to that, they may not even realize that it exists. Between the years of puberty and the mid-forties or so, the gland remains about the size of a walnut, and all is well. But some time during the fifth decade of life, hormonal changes stimulate the prostate gland to grow. And grow. This wouldn't be a problem, except for one pesky little detail. The prostate gland surrounds a very important part of the male anatomy, called the urethra. This pliable, cylindrical tube carries urine from the bladder to its ultimate destination in the outside world. As the doughnut-shaped prostate gland enlarges, the doughnut "hole" gets progressively smaller, squashing the urethra. Once the diameter of a dime, the urethra can become as narrow as a cocktail straw.

This narrowing can cause older men some serious grief, as it dramatically interferes with proper emptying of the bladder. If urine is retained, it could cause a urinary tract infection, which may make intercourse painful. Of course, that doesn't mean that all men with enlarged prostates get urinary tract infections. But it is common for men with this condition to feel the urge to urinate more frequently throughout the day, and even at night. Many men with BPH find it tough to get a decent night's rest because they're up and down all night, trekking back and forth to the bathroom. Just the loss of sleep alone can dampen libido.

While the condition itself is often responsible, the medications used to treat it can be just as problematic. The exact ways in which the enlarged prostate produces misery aren't fully understood, but here's what we do know: Male hormones, including testosterone and its souped-up cousin dihydrotestosterone (DHT), trigger cell growth in the prostate gland. As the gland grows, it begins to put pressure on the urethra.

Although the size of the prostate gland doesn't always correlate with the severity of symptoms, studies show that men who have enlarged prostates are at increased risk for complications, including urinary retention and prostate infections. The good news is that for most men, BPH is a very slow disease process.

Diagnosing and Treating BPH

As the proud owner of a prostate gland, it's important to haul it into the doctor's office every now and then for a checkup. If you're over the age of forty, your doctor may order a blood test called a PSA test, for prostate specific antigen. While PSA level alone isn't enough to distinguish BPH from prostate cancer, it is helpful in some cases. This test helps your doctor evaluate your risk for prostate cancer. A urinalysis is sometimes performed to check for the presence of blood or infection.

Your doctor will undoubtedly evaluate your gland by performing a digital rectal examination (digital meaning finger—gloved in this case; and rectal referring to that part of the anatomy that you'd rather not have a finger anywhere near, gloved or otherwise). Although a rectal examination isn't anyone's idea of a picnic, it's not going to kill you. It's really the only way for your doctor to appreciate the architecture of the gland, by checking for any lumps or bumps that might indicate cancer or infection. If your family doctor detects any abnormalities, he'll undoubtedly want to send you to a urologist for further evaluation, and unfortunately, another rectal exam by another gloved finger. If your symptoms or examination warrant them, the urologist may advise you to undergo further, more invasive tests, including a biopsy of the prostate gland, or having a scope placed in your rectum or bladder to get a bird's eye view of your prostate or bladder. Neither test is especially comfortable or fun, but if they're necessary for your health, you might as well just grin, bend, and bear it.

In a few men with severe cases of BPH, surgery will be absolutely unavoidable. If you've come to the point where surgery seems more appealing than putting up with the unpleasant symptoms of BPH, you'll probably qualify.

In the majority of cases, however, surgery won't be necessary. There are a number of nonoperative BPH treatments available, and if your doctor recommends any one of them, it will probably behoove you to try it. Some treatments involve simple lifestyle changes, and often they bring dramatic results. Avoiding over-the-counter cold and sinus remedies that contain antihistamines is usually helpful. Steering clear of alcohol and coffee after your evening meal will reduce the frequency of your nighttime treks to the bathroom.

For centuries, men have nurtured their prostates with various herbs and plant extracts— saw palmetto is probably the best known. How it works to benefit the prostate gland isn't fully understood, but most experts theorize that its actions include blocking the conversion of testosterone to DHT. Although saw palmetto seems to be totally incapable of shrinking the prostate gland back to its former size, reducing PSA levels, or preventing prostate cancer, several studies have shown that in some men, it is effective in controlling the more annoying symptoms of BPH.

Interestingly, at least two studies have shown an inverse relationship between smoking, alcohol consumption, and the development of BPH. Data from the studies indicated that moderate cigarette smoking and alcohol consumption actually decreased the symptoms of BPH, as well as the risk of requiring prostatic surgery. In spite of these findings, you'll be hard-pressed to find a doctor who recommends taking up drinking and smoking for the greater good of your prostate. Scientists believe that the surprising findings could be due, in part, to the testosterone-lowering effects of alcohol. While this action may have a modest benefit for your prostate gland, it will undoubtedly hamper your sex life. Exercise has been shown to have a protective effect against the symptoms of BPH. Men who walk regularly for exercise have fewer troubling symptoms and require prostate-related surgery less frequently than men with more slug-like exercise habits.

Several prescription medications are available for the treatment of BPH. Those known as alpha-receptor blockers promote the relaxation of the smooth muscles of the bladder and the prostate. This action serves to ease the flow of urine through the urethra. Unfortunately, these medications can also lower your blood pressure to an impressive degree, so you may find yourself feeling a little light-headed or dizzy when you begin using them. With time, these side effects tend to dissipate. Terazosin hydrochloride is a long-acting alpha-blocker that was originally developed as a blood pressure medicine. Side effects are infrequent, but can include dizziness, fainting, and drowsiness. On the plus side, this medication is not likely to alter your sexual function. The long-acting alpha-blocker Doxazosin is similar to Terazosin in actions and side effects, and is usually well-tolerated.

Tamsulosin is an alpha-blocker that acts mainly in the tissues of the prostate gland to reduce symptoms of BPH. Side effects are uncommon, but can include a runny nose, abnormal ejaculation, and dizziness. Drugs known as 5-alpha-reductase inhibitors, including finasteride (Proscar) interfere with the conversion of testosterone to its mischievous cousin, dihydrotestosterone (DHT), a hormone known to be a potent promoter of prostate gland growth. One study indicated that this drug not only alleviates the symptoms of BPH, it may also reduce the risk for complications—and even surgery over the long haul. Side effects of this drug are typically related to sexual function, including problems with ejaculation, decreased libido, and erectile dysfunction. If you and your partner value your sex lives, you might want think long and hard before agreeing to take this one.

PROSTATE CANCER

Ask any man what type of cancer he most fears, and cancer of the prostate gland will rank high on the list. And with good reason—prostate cancer is the most common cancer diagnosed in American men. Each year, more than one hundred and eight thousand American men are diagnosed with the disease, and about thirty-eight thousand will lose their lives to it. If a high PSA level raises the suspicion of cancer, most doctors will recommend a biopsy of the gland, in which a small sample of tissue is removed and examined microscopically for cancerous changes. Tissue biopsies gives patients and their doctors some important information—how aggressive the cancer appears to be, and whether or not it has spread to other parts of the body.

For men with incurable cancer that has escaped the prostate and spread, treatment options are limited. But for men with early cancers that are confined to the prostate, the decision about which treatment to have is a considerably more difficult one to make. In most cases, early prostate cancer is treated with either surgery or radiation therapy. Men who opt for surgery face an operation called a radical prostatectomy, a procedure in which the prostate gland—and hopefully the cancer—is removed from the body. Men who want to avoid surgery can undergo radiation therapy to combat the disease. Although surgery and radiation therapies can deliver a cure, some men feel that the side effects are just as devastating as the disease. Both treatments are associated with the distressing impairment of bladder control, and even worse, the development of sexual dysfunction. Fortunately, the side effects often dissipate with time. In some cases, they can be offset or overcome with prescription medications.

Some experts question whether regular PSA testing leads to unnecessary treatments, especially in elderly men. Skeptics say that there's just not enough evidence to suggest that the PSA test can actually reduce a man's chances of dying from prostate cancer, or that it significantly improves the quality of his life. It is often said that more men die *with* prostate cancer than *from* it. Because most prostate cancers are slow growing, many men are able to live out the remainder of their lives without ever succumbing to the disease. For men whose cancer is found early, it is often difficult to know whether or not treatment is really necessary, and if it is performed, whether or not it will actually work.

The American Urological Association and the American Cancer Society recommend that all men fifty and older consider an annual PSA test along with a yearly digital rectal exam. For men whose family members have had the disease, the test is recommended beginning at the age of forty to forty-five. But currently, the National Cancer Institute makes no specific recommendation about PSA testing.

The decision to undergo testing for prostate cancer may be difficult, but before you decide, be sure to discuss it thoroughly with your doctor. With enough information, the decision you make will be the right one for you.

OBSTRUCTIVE SLEEP APNEA

If your snoring has driven your bedfellow to quieter sleeping quarters, more than your relationship could be at stake. Snoring is a red flag for a more serious condition known as obstructive sleep apnea (OSA), a condition marked by diminished airflow to the lungs during sleep. Testosterone is known to be influential in the onset and worsening of the condition, and as a result, men are much more likely to develop the condition than are women. Obstructive sleep apnea is most often diagnosed in obese, middle-aged men with high blood pressure. Unless they're morbidly obese, women rarely develop the condition before menopause.

Almost everyone experiences brief episodes of sleep apnea, a period in which breathing momentarily stops during slumber, but an estimated two to five million Americans stop breathing several hundred times each night, for periods of time ranging from ten seconds to more than two minutes. Fortunately, most people wake up before they die, but to stop breathing is still quite hazardous to their health. While you sleep, the muscles of your pharynx, or throat, become slack, making your airways more susceptible to collapse and blockage. The presence of any abnormal structure in your airways makes you much more susceptible to the development of sleep apnea. Obstructive sleep apnea can be caused by growths in the nasal passageways called nasal polyps, or by a deviated septum, in which the nasal passages are crooked. In the mouth and throat, an enlarged tongue or tonsils may be the culprit, but in most cases, obesity is at the root of the problem.

As we gain weight, fat accumulates almost everywhere in the body. Most of us are painfully aware of the fat deposits that pile up in double and triple chins, but fat is also stored in the cells of your nose and throat. With a little help from gravitational forces, these fat stores can compress the airways of your upper respiratory tract by virtue of their sheer weight, effectively halting the flow of air to your lungs, causing your blood oxygen to plummet to a critically low level. Your heart rate, which may normally trip along at about seventy to eighty beats per minute, can slow to a dangerous thirty beats per minute. In response to this type of asphyxia, and the impending death it represents, your body pushes the panic button. Your brain saves your life by instructing you to wake up, open your mouth, and breathe. You may have narrowly escaped death, but even more hazardous events await you. Upon re-breathing, your heart races, often to the dangerous tune of more than 120 beats per minute. For susceptible folk, this rapid heart rate can trigger abnormal heart rhythms, which can lead to an entirely separate set of problems. If you survive the heart-racing episode unscathed, your slumber will resume, and chances are good that you'll never even know about your close call. Incredibly, this traumatic sequence of events can be repeated hundreds of times every single night. Although you may not be consciously aware of your frequent awakenings, the constant interruptions in your sleep will eventually take their toll. People with OSA experience profound daytime sleepiness, fatigue, and impaired concentration.

Not everyone who snores qualifies for the diagnosis of OSA, but snoring is a good indication that you have the condition. Snoring results from the high frequency vibration of the tissues in the mouth and throat. This vibration is so extreme that it actually traumatizes the involved tissues, creating swelling and causing the airways to narrow even more.

Most OSA sufferers seek help for one of two reasons. Some go to their doctors voluntarily when chronic sleep deprivation leads to sleep apnea syndrome, a condition that plagues men twice as often as women. Initially marked by morning sluggishness, sleep apnea syndrome progresses to daytime fatigue and a complete inability to stay awake. Impairment of memory, judgment, and concentration soon follow. At some point, OSA sufferers frequently develop trouble in their relationships. Lack of sleep can lead to significant personality changes, and it can totally wipe out libido. In severe cases, it can lead to erectile dysfunction. Those OSA sufferers who don't seek medical attention for themselves will often cave in after their significant others threaten them with abandonment. Bedfellows of the OSA-afflicted typically describe their partners' snoring as loud and rhythmic, punctuated by long periods of breathless silence and followed by loud snorts, or gasps. Snorers are known to thrash wildly about the bed, often inflicting bodily injury on their partners.

If you have OSA, your bed partner can probably make the diagnosis, but it is still important to seek medical attention. Your doctor will want to conduct a thorough search of your nose and throat for signs of narrowing or obstruction. If you've got a little extra cash and some nice pajamas, you might want to submit yourself to a sleep study. The test is expensive and time consuming, but in most cases, it is completely necessary. For about $1,200-to-$1,500, you'll be treated to a one-night stay in a sleep clinic, during which time your brain activity, blood oxygen level, and heart rate are monitored while you sleep. If the sleep study confirms the diagnosis of OSA, your first course of action will be to lose weight, and fortunately, this measure is often curative. Your doctor will undoubtedly invite you to avoid alcohol, especially around bedtime. Even a nightcap or two can cause sleep apnea in otherwise healthy people. Obstructive sleep apnea is sometimes treated using dental appliances. Wearing a specially designed mouthpiece while you sleep helps hold your jaw forward and prevents collapse of the airways. While they're relatively effective, most people find them uncomfortable and unromantic, and many refuse to wear them on a regular basis. Since lying on your back exacerbates OSA, you'll be instructed to sleep on your side or stomach. If you've been sleeping in the same position for several decades, this is easier said than done. You can discourage back-sleeping by sewing tennis balls on the back of your favorite jammies, or you can try wearing a fanny pack stuffed with a hard plastic object, like a hairbrush. Your bed partner will probably be delighted to assist you in the design of the appropriate device.

If you have a serious case of OSA, your doctor will recommend that you use a machine that delivers pressurized oxygen to your airways via a mask. This device, called a CPAP (continuous positive airway pressure) machine, can help hold airways open during sleep and prevent OSA. This treatment is very effective while it's used, but about a quarter of people who are pre-scribed CPAP machines find them intolerable. If all else fails, an operation called uvulopalatopharyngoplasty, or UPPP, may be your last chance at a cure. This surgical procedure consists of an amputation of the uvula, the gooey stalactite at the back of your throat, as well as a small portion of the soft palate in your mouth. This procedure is not pain free, by any means, but it does provide a cure to about half of the people who choose to have it done.

In spite of all that modern medicine has to offer, most people with OSA are not cured, and the goal of treatment is simply to control their symptoms. Obstructive sleep apnea and its complications usually progress with age. When it occasionally occurs, death from OSA usually results from the development of irregular heart rhythms and heart attacks; complications of high blood pressure; or by automobile accidents caused by dozing off at the wheel. To date, there are no reported deaths at the hands of a frustrated bed-fellow, and you certainly won't want to be the first one to achieve this dubious honor. When it comes to your overall health, and especially your sexuality, treatment of OSA can make a world of difference.

VASECTOMY

The decision to permanently remove yourself from the gene pool is a difficult one. But given the surprisingly high number of babies born to couples using temporary means of contraception, sterilization can be an attractive option. And women aren't the only ones going under the knife—more men are deciding to have vasectomies. A vasectomy is a procedure in which the male "tubes" are tied. The tubes themselves—the vas defera—are a pair of eighteen-inch long structures that carry sperm out of the testes. Vasectomies usually involve making two small cuts in the upper part of the scrotum. Working through these openings, the doctor finds the tubes, cuts them, and ties the ends. The entire procedure takes less than half an hour, start to finish.

It's hard for men to believe, but vasectomies are actually considered to be rather minor surgical procedures. They're also extremely safe. In the United States, where nearly 500,000 vasectomies are performed every year, there have been no reported deaths associated with the procedure itself. And complications are rare, occurring in less than 1 percent of patients.

While traditional vasectomies have been performed successfully for over a century, a relatively new procedure, called the "no-scalpel vasectomy" is gaining popularity. In this operation, the tubes are tied through two tiny holes in the scrotum, making it even quicker, safer, and less painful. About one third of all vasectomies in the U.S. are performed using this method. Regardless of the type of procedure employed, vasectomies are usually performed in a surgical office with the patient fully awake, but rendered nearly pain-free with a local anesthetic. Most men experience temporary discomfort after the procedure, and swelling and bruising in the area aren't uncommon. An ice pack, a few pain pills, and a day or two of rest will usually take care of the pain and swelling. In a week to ten days, most guys are back to normal and ready to take on their regular activities.

No matter what you've heard, a vasectomy doesn't affect any aspect of your manhood except your ability to father children. The chances that you'll suddenly develop a high-pitched voice or a beehive hairdo are virtually nil. Having a vasectomy has no measurable effect on weight gain, libido, semen production, or testosterone levels. There's no link between vasectomy and testicular cancer. Although some studies have found a slightly higher rate of prostate cancer in men who have had vasectomies, no one knows for sure if the two are actually related. Some experts believe that men with vasectomies don't really have a higher rate of prostate cancer, they just have a higher rate of detection. Since these men are more likely to visit doctors than other men, they're more likely to have their prostate cancers discovered.

Vasectomies are extremely effective in the long run, but results aren't immediate. It can take up to six months after the surgery before you're completely sterile, so it's important to take precautions until your doctor gives you the all clear. A year after your surgery, the chance that your tubes will grow back together is about one in twenty-three hundred. If you've had a vasectomy, you can be proud. Surveys show that most men who have the procedure are highly intelligent, responsible, and secure in their masculinity. And more importantly, they're much less likely to be handing out cigars in the middle of the night.

TESTICULAR CANCER

Although testicular cancer accounts for less than 2 percent of all cancers in men, it's the most common cancer to strike young men, especially those between the ages of fifteen and thirty-four. Each year, over seven thousand American men will be diagnosed with the disease. The incidence of testicular cancer in the United States has almost doubled since the 1930s, and the numbers are continuing to climb. The good news is that although more men are being diagnosed with the cancer, fewer are dying from it, thanks to better treatments.

The risk of testicular cancer is highest in white men, especially those who have family members with the disease. For some reason, men of African descent are rarely affected. About 10 percent of testicular tumors are diagnosed in men with a history of a testicle that failed to descend normally. When this condition is found in boys, it is almost always surgically corrected. But even after correction, the risk of testicular cancer is almost ten times greater than in men who didn't have the condition.

Although many men diagnosed with testicular cancer report a recent injury to the affected testicle, doctors don't believe there's really any relationship between injury and the disease. Men with injuries are more likely to examine their testicles, and may notice lumps and bumps while they're at it. There doesn't seem to be any correlation between testicular cancer and occupational exposures or sports participation, either. If you are diagnosed with the disease, your doctor will undoubtedly recommend that you have surgery to remove the affected testicle.

It's not something that anyone looks forward to, but in most cases, the surgery is a lifesaver. Occasionally, radiation or chemotherapy will also be necessary. The good news is that in many cases, the remaining testicle is healthy and fully functional, and is capable of producing adequate levels of testosterone to keep your libido intact.

ANDROPAUSE

Although a great deal is understood about female menopause, comparatively little is known about the male equivalent, called "andropause." In women, drastic reductions in levels of the hormone estrogen trigger the well-defined symptoms of menopause. In men, andropause occurs as the result of dwindling levels of testosterone. But while estrogen levels take a hard nosedive in middle-aged women, the decline in male testosterone production is slow and progressive, making the symptoms of andropause harder to recognize in aging men.

Starting at the tender age of forty, testosterone production in men begins to drop at a rate of about 1 percent per year. By the time men are in their sixties, testosterone levels may have fallen to below-normal levels. Low levels of testosterone can bring about subtle changes. Like menopausal women, andropausal men can experience hot flashes, irritability, trouble concentrating, and insomnia. Many men notice a lighter beard growth and sparser body hair, as well as the accumulation of body fat and loss of muscle mass. Left untreated, low testosterone levels can deplete bone mass, leading to osteoporosis and bone fractures. For many men, the most disturbing symptom of andropause is a noticeable decline in libido, and in some cases, the warning signs of sexual dysfunction.

Treatment for Andropause

While the symptoms of andropause are real and potentially hazardous to male health, most andropausal men don't receive treatment—much less testing—for the condition. An estimated four to five million American men are running low on testosterone, but fewer than two-hundred thousand are currently being treated. This lack of medical attention can be blamed in part on a serious lag in medical knowledge. Some experts believe that gradually declining testosterone levels in aging men are natural, and even protective. Most doctors aren't entirely sure whether they should replace dwindling hormone levels with testosterone replacement therapy, or simply sit back and let nature take its course.

There's good reason for the confusion. Studies looking at testosterone replacement therapy in aging men have generated mixed results. While men receiving supplemental testosterone show significant gains in muscle and bone mass, less body fat, and dramatic improvements in energy levels and moods, testosterone replacement therapy isn't entirely risk-free. In older men, testosterone supplementation has been shown to trigger benign growth of the prostate gland and unmask prostate cancer. It can aggravate sleep apnea, which in turn increases the risk of heart disease.

At a recent meeting of The Endocrine Society however, male hormone replacement therapy with low dose testosterone was pronounced safe and effective. This finding was based, in part, on the results of an ongoing study performed at the University Chicago Medical School. The authors studied the beneficial effects and safety of low-dose testosterone replacement therapy in healthy men aged sixty-five to eighty-five. Compared with other healthy middle-aged males, the subjects' baseline levels of free testosterone were determined to be "borderline low." Beginning in 1993, the men received intra-muscular injections of testosterone, either twenty-five milligrams a week or fifty milligrams every two weeks. During the study, testosterone levels increased, but there was no change noted in liver enzymes or incidence of sleep apnea. Testosterone replacement therapy had significant benefits in terms of lipid metabolism, osteoporosis, muscle mass, fat distribution, libido, and mood. There were no adverse effects reported. The authors concluded that in low doses, supplemental testosterone is safe for the male heart and circulatory system, as well as the prostate gland. It also seems to play an important role in the prevention of osteoporosis in men.

While there is still a great deal of controversy about whether or not to treat andropausal men with supplemental testosterone, one thing is clear. Hormonal replacement therapy for men has never been simpler. In the past, men who required supplemental testosterone had only one option: testosterone injections. The shots, given once every three to four weeks, are effective, safe, and only a little bit painful. At a cost of about ten dollars per dose, the medicine itself is very inexpensive. The downside to testosterone injections is that hormone levels tend to fall precipitously between doses, resulting in the recurrence of symptoms.

Over the past decade, several new testosterone replacement therapies have become available. Testoderm, available since 1994, is a hormone-impregnated patch that is applied to the shaved skin of the scrotum. The thin skin in this area allows for easy absorption of the medication into the bloodstream. A small percentage of men who wear the patch experience itching and skin irritation, but these symptoms usually diminish with time. The cost of the patch is around $90 for a month's supply. Another testosterone patch, Androderm, has been on the market since 1995. The patch has the distinct advantage of being suitable for application to the skin of the abdomen, upper arm, or thigh. The downside to using this product is that nearly half of all men using it experience skin reactions, some of which are quite severe.

The newest testosterone replacement product approved by the Food and Drug Administration is AndroGel, a testosterone gel that can be rubbed onto the skin of the abdomen, upper arm, or shoulder. AndroGel may be the easiest product to use, but its convenience comes at a higher price: A month's supply can set you back about $150. Since all testosterone replacement therapy options are effective, choosing one over the others comes down to individual preference, convenience, and cost. The most important decision to be made is whether or not to use the products at all.

CHAPTER 8

IS YOUR PRESCRIPTION DRUG TO BLAME?

IN CASE ANYONE'S COUNTING, THERE ARE AN ESTIMATED TWO HUNDRED DRUGS on the market today that have been found to have a direct impact on sexuality. In most instances, that impact isn't exactly favorable. These medicines can leave men with serious erectile problems, cause sexual arousal disorder in women, and lack-luster libido in both. Experts speculate that of the 90 percent of cases of sexual dysfunction that can be traced to a physical cause, at least a quarter of these can be attributed to a drug of some sort.

Often the sexual problems related to medications aren't discussed at the time your doctor prescribes them, nor are they highlighted—or even mentioned—in the package inserts that accompany the drugs. There are a number of explanations for this. For starters, pharmaceutical companies may not have your best sexual interests at heart. In clinical trials, they rarely make a point of asking volunteers taking the drugs about their products' sexual side effects—they're more concerned with "important" side effects, like nausea, diarrhea, or constipation. It's understandable that most subjects wouldn't be all that comfortable volunteering information relating to their sub-par sexual performance, so many reports of sexual side effects never make it to consumers. Because you may not be advised to look for sexual side effects, it will take a little detective work on your behalf to discover whether or not the drugs you're taking are interfering with your sexual health in any way.

Although some drug companies have had the foresight and courtesy to report the sexual side effects of their drugs in men, they have neglected to discuss any unintended sexual outcomes in women. This may be due to the fact that unfavorable sexual outcomes in men are more visibly apparent than those in women, and women may be less apt to report any adverse sexual effects. Women shouldn't hesitate to tell their physicians about any drug-related sexual side effects, including vaginal dryness, general lack of libido, decreased breast or genital sensation, or lack of responsiveness. Since the physiology of sex and the sexual response cycle aren't fully understood in the first place, most doctors, scientists, and pharmacists can hardly claim to completely appreciate the potential sexual side effects of any medication. Don't hesitate to speak up and stick to your guns, and ask your physician to work with you. It's possible that your doctor can immediately reverse the problem by changing the dose, or the medication itself.

When it comes to prescription medications, the most common sex offenders can be grouped according to the classes listed below.

- *Antacids,* used to treat stomach ulcers, gastroesophageal reflux, and other gastronomic maladies: Tagamet, Pepcid, Prilosec, Zantac
- *Anti-alcohol drugs,* used to treat alcoholism: Antabuse
- *Antibiotics,* almost any type, but especially broad-spectrum antibiotics used to treat infections of the respiratory tract, urinary tract, skin, and gastrointestinal system. These drugs can change the natural vaginal flora in women, resulting in vaginal yeast infections and irritation, as well as discomfort with intercourse.
- *Anticholesterol drugs,* used to treat high cholesterol and high triglyceride levels: Lopid
- *Antiepileptic drugs,* used to treat seizure disorders, migraine headaches, tics, and chronic pain disorders: Dilantin
- *Antifungal drugs,* used to treat fungal infections of the skin, nails, and other body parts: Nizoral
- *Antihistamines,* found in numerous over-the-counter and prescription medications to treat symptoms of the common cold, sinus problems, allergies, and motion sickness. These substances can dry the mucous membranes in the respiratory tract, an action that is helpful in alleviating the symptoms of allergies. But this medication effect can also dry the mucous membranes of the vagina, an action that will interfere with lubrication. Some of the older antihistamines, including Benadryl and Chlor-Trimeton can impair the part of the nervous system that is crucial to sexual response. In some susceptible individuals,

these drugs can inhibit arousal and prevent orgasm. They may also numb the mind and the senses, and cause drowsiness; both effects can make foreplay a frustrating affair. Newer allergy medicines, like Claritin and Allegra, don't seem to have the same types of side effects. Taking them may help alleviate your itchy nose and watery eyes, and still allow you to have enjoyable sex.

- *Antihypertensives*, used to lower blood pressure and treat heart disease, and occasionally used to treat headaches and other medical conditions. These drugs can affect the central nervous system, altering levels of neurotransmitters, like dopamine, that are critical in the sexual response cycle. They may also impair genital sensation and impede the rapid flow of blood to the pelvis that normally occurs during arousal. These include:

  Diuretics, sometimes referred to as "water" pills or "fluid" pills, are often used to treat high blood pressure, bloating or swelling, and heart disease. Diuretics may interfere with sexuality through their zinc-depleting actions, which in turn allows the body to more freely transform testosterone into estrogen. This phenomenon may ultimately have libido-lowering effects in roughly a third of the men and women who use them.

  Spironolactone, a medicine primarily used to treat fluid retention and hypertension, is known to block the action of testosterone. With this in mind, doctors often prescribe it to treat acne and unwanted hair growth in women. Its testosterone-dampening actions have long been associated with libido-lowering effects and erection disturbances.

  Medications that fall into the **"beta-blocker"** family of drugs, including Inderal, Lopressor, Tenormin, as well as a whole smorgasbord of generic copycats, are often guilty of interfering with sexuality. These drugs are commonly used to lower blood pressure and treat heart disease, and in many cases, can help prevent heart attacks and prolong life. On the downside, they're notorious for causing fatigue, an action that may leave you too tired to engage in sexual activity. They're also known to cause problems with erection in men and sexual arousal in women.

  Clonidine, a drug used to control high blood pressure, has been shown to cause erectile dysfunction in men. In animal studies, it regularly reduces blood flow to the penis and diminishes the volume of the subjects' ejaculations. In male rats, it suppresses sexual activity and prevents ejaculation. Female rats receiving the drug display a noticeable lack of sexually receptive behavior, even in the presence of undeniably attractive males. If your doctor feels that your very survival depends on taking this drug, you might want to inquire about the safety of taking yohimbine along with it. Several studies have demonstrated that yohimbine blocks most of Clonidine's antisexual side effects.

- *Anti-inflammatory agents*, used to treat the pain and inflammation of conditions like arthritis, headaches, and menstrual pain. Anaprox, Naprosyn, and their generic equivalents are the greatest offenders.
- *Antiestablishment drugs*, used primarily in the pursuit of an altered states of consciousness. Marijuana, cocaine, heroin, and ecstasy are commonly used in the U.S. While regular users of marijuana say that the weed has positive impacts on libido and sexual performance, it is quite possible that they are mistaken. After all, marijuana use is known to impair judgment and memory. And, since possessing and partaking of marijuana for any reason are still considered criminal activities in most parts of the U.S., it's hard to justify its use. Most scientific studies show that over the long haul, chronic use of marijuana is detrimental to both sexual interest and sexual performance.

  While use of illicit drugs that are considered to be uppers, like cocaine and heroin, may initially boost energy levels and create feelings of euphoria, the "crash" that follows (not to mention the potential jail time) will definitely kill the mood. Use of these drugs will undoubtedly prove to be dangerous, if not deadly.

- *Antianxiety or anxiolytic drugs* used to treat disorders of anxiety and panic, and occasionally seizures. They include Valium, Xanax, and Klonopin. Any tranquilizer or antianxiety drug is capable of disrupting normal sexual function. For starters, these types of medications can dramatically dull your senses and bring on sleep, even in the most sexually provocative situations. At one time or another, most users have reported unpleasant side effects associated with the use of these drugs, including decreased libido, sedation and drowsiness, and a generalized state of muscle relaxation so profound that it can cause the entire body to feel limp. In one study of the drug Klonopin, 90 percent of users were found to experience negative sexual side effects.

If you can taper off these medicines and still survive your life, you might want to consider it. Your sex life will probably flourish. If stopping your medication is simply out of the question, you might be able to get by with either a lower dose, or less frequent dosing.

- *Analgesic drugs,* commonly prescribed for short periods of time to treat acute pain, such as narcotics like Lortab and Percocet; and barbiturates, including Butalbital and Esgic. Both classes of drugs can lead to sexual dysfunction in men and women.

- *Amphetamines,* occasionally used to treat attention deficit disorder in adults. Ritalin is the one most commonly prescribed.

- *Appetite suppressants,* commonly used to treat overeating and obesity, include Meridia, a serotonin reuptake inhibitor, which was originally developed as an antidepressant medication. Like the other antidepressants in the SSRI class, Meridia's side effects include diminished libido and delayed orgasm. Other appetite-suppressing drugs, including Fastin, Adipex, and their generic equivalents, are actually amphetamines. In susceptible people, these drugs are known to cause increased heart rate, nervousness, irritability, and sexual dysfunction. Men taking one of these drugs may experience trouble getting or maintaining erections. If you value your sex life, you might want to forego the pills and try to lose weight the old-fashioned way, with a healthy diet and plenty of exercise.

- *Antidepressants,* used to treat depression. Several classes of antidepressant drugs can interfere dramatically with libido, arousal, and sexual performance in men and women. Selective serotonin reuptake inhibitors (SSRIs) are currently recognized as the drugs of choice for the treatment of depressive disorders. These drugs are extremely popular with both physicians and their patients because they are easy to take, well-tolerated, and have excellent safety profiles. These drugs work by blocking the "reuptake" and subsequent breakdown of serotonin, increasing the concentration of this "feel-good" neurotransmitter in the central nervous system. The SSRIs are incredibly versatile drugs, and are often prescribed to treat conditions other than depression, including anxiety and panic disorders, social phobia, obsessive compulsive disorder, chronic pain, and premenstrual dysphoric disorder.

  Prozac (fluoxetine) was the first SSRI drug to be approved by the FDA for the treatment of depression. In the decades that followed, the list of

SSRIs has grown to include Zoloft (sertraline), Paxil (paroxetine), Celexa (Citalopram), Luvox (fluvoxamine), and Lexapro (escitalopram). Although the drugs share a similar mechanism of action, the structural differences among them leaves each medication with a different set of side effects and drug interactions. All things considered, the SSRI drugs are commonly associated with side effects that include transient nausea, diarrhea, insomnia, drowsiness, dizziness, diminished libido, and long-term orgasmic dysfunction.

One rather novel antidepressant, called **Effexor** (venlafaxine) has a mechanism of action similar to the SSRIs, but it has the additional effect of blocking the breakdown of norepinephrine, a neurotransmitter that has been implicated in depression. Its side effects, including those involving sexual response and performance, are similar to the SSRI drugs'.

While the SSRI antidepressants and their chemical cousin, Effexor, have undoubtedly made millions of folks feel better by alleviating symptoms of depression, the widespread Prozac-ation of America may have a lot to do with the sorry state of sexual affairs in our great nation.

If you and your doctor agree that you need to take an SSRI to stay on an even emotional keel, you can still salvage your sex life by trying one of several approaches. First, you can try to reduce the dose. It's entirely possible that you may feel just as well on a dose that is a little lower. Some doctors advocate taking what they call a "sex-and-drug" holiday. Antidepressant-induced sexual dysfunction typically reverses within one to three days after stopping the drug. Likewise, you can expect to experience the sexual side effects within one to three days after restarting the drug. To prepare for your exciting sex and drug holiday, you'll be advised to stop taking your medication for a few days, during which time you will hopefully experience an incredibly fulfilling sexual encounter. This type of approach definitely squashes any type of sexual spontaneity, but you can overcome this problem simply by planning to be spontaneous in advance.

If neither of these approaches works, or if you're not exactly crazy about trying them in the first place, there are still other options. Your doctor may advise you to change medications completely. You'll likely be offered a drug that belongs in a different class than the SSRIs. The antidepressant Wellbutrin (bupropion) has earned a reputation as a sexuality-sparing drug, and most folks find that it not only allows them to return to their normal levels of libido and sexual performance, but it also effectively treats their depressive symptoms.

In some cases, sexual side effects may be alleviated simply by adding a dose of Wellbutrin to the antidepressant medication that you're currently taking. Some doctors prescribe other medicines to help their patients overcome the sexual side effects of antidepressants, including Periactin (cyproheptadine), a medication used to treat allergies; Serzone (nefazodone), an antidepressant; and Remeron (mirtazapine) a so-called "tetracycline" antidepressant. In many cases, a properly timed dose of Viagra may be all it takes to restore erectile function. While Viagra may improve sexual performance, it is not known to enhance libido, a very necessary component of sexuality.

It's never a good idea to abruptly abandon your medications in the interest of salvaging your sex life. You certainly won't want to risk having a major panic attack, stroke, or heart attack, or worsen any existing medical conditions. On the other hand, it's important for you, and especially for your doctor, to remember that good sexual health is often critical to your overall well-being. If a medicine lowers your blood pressure like a champ, but makes it difficult to enjoy sex in any way, then maybe it's not such a great drug after all. Unless your doctor has a fully functional crystal ball, there's no way she'll know about the sexual side effects you happen to experience with the drug she prescribes, so it's absolutely essential that you volunteer the information. Most doctors are more than happy to adjust your medications in hopes of allowing you to continue to enjoy your sexuality to the hilt. In the meantime, ask your doctor about nonpharmaceutical methods of improving your condition. Sometimes, a few changes in the diet and exercise departments might be all that are necessary to improve your physical health and eliminate your need for the drug in the first place.

PART III

CHAPTER 9

SEX ON THE BRAIN

SEXUAL DESIRE IS ALL IN YOUR HEAD—LITERALLY. The human brain is ultimately behind every thought, every movement, and every physiological response that encompasses the process of making love. A single erotic thought or sexual fantasy can spark desire and trigger a complex cascade of events that leads to arousal. The brain's power over the body's sexual response is of such magnitude that it is entirely possible for human beings to experience orgasm in the total absence of any external stimulation—not that this is always a good thing, but it's interesting to contemplate the notion that it all starts with a single, simple thought.

Although we usually tend to think of "thoughts" as abstract products of our nebulous "minds," we need to get a bit more technical about the whole concept in order to understand the brain's role in sexuality. In scientific terms, thoughts are tiny electrical impulses that travel through the human brain, delivering signals from one point to another. These impulses are carried along on the coattails of brain chemicals called neurotransmitters. While there are undoubtedly dozens—or even hundreds—of neurotransmitters that have managed to elude scientific discovery, a few have been thoroughly studied and are reasonably well-understood. Several of them are known to play critical roles in human sexuality.

Neurotransmitters exert their influence in both direct and indirect ways. In the short run, they are directly responsible for creating the emotional desire and longing for sexual activity and the physical state necessary to engage in it. Over the long haul, they are the substances that create moods, attitudes, and beliefs that indirectly determine many aspects of our sexuality. Neurotransmitters allow us to derive enjoyment from sex on several levels: biochemically, emotionally, and physically. Without the complex interplay of these chemicals in the brain, sex might end up being just another bodily function. Understanding the roles that the various neurotransmitters play in human sexuality is important. The more you know about them, the better your ability to capitalize on their actions. To some degree, you can even learn to manipulate their levels to optimize your sexual desire, performance, and enjoyment.

The production, release, and regulation of neurotransmitters are ultimately dependent upon your diet and your lifestyle. The foods that you eat on a daily basis provide the substrates for the manufacture of brain chemicals. If your diet doesn't contain a wide variety of wholesome foods, you are depriving your body of the nutrients it needs to create the neurotransmitters that are vital to emotional and sexual health. Overloading your body with excessive salt, sugar, caffeine, and fat is not only bad for your body; it also disrupts the precise balance of neurochemicals in your brain. While eating a nutritious, well balanced diet is critical, *when* you eat is almost as important as *what* you eat. In order to provide your brain with a steady supply of the necessary nutrients, you must eat regularly throughout the day.

Stress management is critical to optimizing neurotransmitter production and regulation. Although many people rely on alcohol and cigarettes to unwind, excessive use of either substance actually compounds the negative effects of stress. If you don't have a healthy, detoxifying outlet for your tension, stress-related hormones like cortisol and adrenaline accumulate and wreak havoc on your emotional and physical health, and ultimately your sexuality. Proper stress management includes getting an adequate amount of sleep and plenty of regular exercise. Nurturing your body is vital to your physical, emotional, and sexual health. A little dietary discretion, combined with a healthy mix of rest and exercise will go a long way toward optimizing your brain's neurochemical balance and enhancing your sexuality.

DOPAMINE

Dopamine is a key neurotransmitter in your brain, and it plays a starring role in sexuality. It allows you to respond to the delightful and provocative messages delivered by your senses, heightening your receptivity and responsiveness to sexual stimulation. Ultimately, it is the neurotransmitter that is responsible for generating the intense rush of pleasure that occurs with orgasm.

Given the profound pleasure generated by the release of dopamine in the brain, it isn't too farfetched to think that the dopamine reward system might have played a crucial role in evolution. The neurotransmitter provides powerful, positive feedback whenever creatures engage in life-affirming behaviors—especially those that help ensure the survival of their species. Elevated levels of dopamine have been associated with eating nutrient-dense foods, with risk-taking behaviors, and with the act of sexual intercourse. If you think about it, these behaviors were obviously useful to our prehistoric ancestors. Eating calorie-dense foods during times of plenty made it possible to survive during periods when food was scarce. In harsh environments, taking risks could mean the difference between life and death. Engaging in sexual intercourse helped ensure a fresh crop of newcomers in the next generation.

While these behaviors were life- and species-sustaining for our ancestors, nowadays we've pretty much outgrown them. In modern societies, they're not nearly as useful as they were a few millennia ago, and, in many cases, they're disastrously counterproductive. Now that food is plentiful, the dopamine-driven indulgence in high-calorie foods has resulted in a worldwide epidemic of obesity. Individuals hooked on the dopamine kick that comes from engaging in risky behaviors are known to develop all kinds of afflictions, ranging from gambling addiction to compulsive shopping. The dopamine-derived high that follows sexual intercourse has contributed to global overpopulation.

Laboratory studies help demonstrate the lengths to which creatures will go to activate the dopamine reward system. In an experiment in which rats were able to push levers to stimulate dopamine release in their brains, they literally died of ecstasy. Pleasure-seeking rats pressed the levers continually, without pausing even to eat. Sadly, they ended up dying of starvation, although apparently in a state of total bliss.

Like the rats in the study, people are only too willing to make huge sacrifices in exchange for a dopamine kick. Throughout history, creative men and women have discovered and engineered dozens of bizarre methods designed to exploit the dopamine reward system. Through trial and error, we've found that it's not all that difficult to score a major dopamine rush from all kinds of substances and activities. Most of them have nothing to do with the survival of our species, and many are decidedly detrimental to our survival. Consumption of alcohol, cocaine, nicotine, chocolate, and even the experience of severe pain can all push the button that delivers the dopamine rush.

In its constant pursuit of homeostasis, or a steady state of being, the human body has found ways to manage these excesses of pleasure, and restore its natural internal balance. In the presence of perpetually high levels of dopamine, the brain begins to reduce the number of dopamine-binding sites on its resident nerve cells. Unable to latch onto the appropriate nerves, the unattached dopamine is powerless to stimulate the pleasure centers of the brain. This phenomenon helps explains why addicts find themselves in need of more frequent "fixes" in ever-higher doses to achieve the same degree of pleasure. Eventually, the protective down-regulation of dopamine receptors leaves the brain in a state of burnout. Addicts often find themselves incapable of experiencing satisfaction—much less bliss—even when life-threatening or lethal doses of the favored substance are consumed.

Fortunately, there's really no need to resort to taking illicit substances or engaging in bizarre behaviors to experience a natural high from dopamine. Having great sex with your lover is an excellent way to trigger the dopamine rush without many of the associated risks. While engaging in sexual activity has a powerful effect on dopamine levels, levels of dopamine in the brain, in turn, have powerful effects on sexuality.

Eating protein rich foods, exercising, and taking the amino acid supplements arginine and tyrosine are also known to boost brain levels of dopamine, and they may add a little more zest to your sex life.

NOREPINEPHRINE

Norepinephrine, also called noradrenaline, is a neurotransmitter that is chemically similar to dopamine. Both are made in the brain from the same basic material: tyrosine, an amino acid that is obtained from foods in your diet. Like dopamine, norepinephrine drives sexual behavior and improves mood. While the neurotransmitter is important for emotional health, it is also important for physical well-being. It plays a role in the fight-or-flight response triggered by stress, and in the normal function of the immune system. Norepinephrine boosts memory, learning, and concentration.

When norepinephrine levels fall below normal, depression may result.

Without the mood-enhancing and motivational effects supplied by this neurotransmitter, individuals may become apathetic, lethargic, and depressed. Several antidepressant drugs, including the tricyclic antidepressants and the antidepressant drug, Effexor, work by increasing norepinephrine levels in the brain.

Without the protective actions of norepinephrine, human beings are vulnerable to the harmful emotional and physical effects of stress. When stress is ongoing, norepinephrine is depleted, which in turn, leaves the immune system less able to fend off minor illnesses and even major diseases. Individuals who are chronically stressed are more susceptible to depression, the common cold, and even cancer.

In large part, norepinephrine is responsible for sex drive. It promotes the emotional states that are conducive to lovemaking, and is the primary neurotransmitter used by the nervous system to trigger sexual interest and activity. It also helps regulate sexual behavior by stimulating the release of hormones that regulate sex drive, and generates the positive moods and emotions that are conducive to lovemaking.

OXYTOCIN

Oxytocin is probably best known for its role in inducing labor and lactation in women. Until recently, this hormone/neurotransmitter wasn't credited with much else. But the influence of oxytocin goes much deeper than just triggering physical processes like uterine contractions and the secretion of breast milk. It is also responsible for cementing what is undeniably the most solid and loving relationship known to human beings: the bond that exists between a mother and her child.

When a woman nurses her newborn, surges of oxytocin in her brain trigger profound emotional changes. Many new mothers report feeling a depth of love and a sense of connection that they had never imagined possible. While oxytocin triggers the "letdown" of breast milk and nurturing behaviors in the mother, it also works to solidify the infant's love for his mother. In response to nursing, infants release their own oxytocin. Under the spell of this powerful hormone, mother and child meld together, gaze deep into each other's eyes, and experience indescribable feelings of love and closeness.

Fortunately, nursing mothers and their babies don't have a corner on the oxytocin market. The hormone is produced and released by children and adults of all ages, at every stage of life. It is now generally accepted that oxytocin exerts a powerful influence on all types of bonding behaviors, serving as the love glue for our most intimate relationships.

While the mouth-to-breast contact of nursing triggers oxytocin release in the brain, it is also secreted in response to many other forms of stimulation. Touch can elicit oxytocin secretion. Studies have demonstrated elevated oxytocin levels in subjects who are receiving neck and shoulder massages. I haven't conducted any formal studies, but I have observed some interesting human behaviors in response to touch. Many of my patients frequent a local hair salon that employs a quiet, unassuming middle-aged man as a shampooer. His job is to shampoo the heads of the women patrons before escorting them to their respective hairstylists. He is undoubtedly very skilled at his trade, but that's not what sets him apart from many of his counterparts in other salons.

At the start of each shampoo session, the man sets a timer, and for five full minutes, women are treated to a luxurious scalp and neck massage. Not only do the women have very clean hair at the end of their shampoo sessions, but they also report feeling incredibly relaxed, overcome with feelings of goodwill, and in many cases, even turned on.

It's important to point out that by current standards, the shampoo man doesn't really qualify as a certifiable hunk. Nor is he a brilliant conversationalist—in fact, he rarely says more than a few words to his female clients. Yet interestingly, this man has an incredible female following and a near legendary local reputation. Women talk about the shampoo man in terms that would make any man's heart and head swell with pride. What they *don't* talk about are his dashing good looks, his sparkling sense of humor, his awesome physical attributes, or any of the run-of-the-mill aspects of manhood that are typically considered to be of supreme importance to the opposite sex. What the women *do* talk about is how the shampoo man makes them *feel*. In the space of five short minutes, using nothing more than scalp-to-finger contact, this man manages to totally recreate his clients' emotional states.

While visual and verbal stimulation are undoubtedly important to human sexuality, the power of touch and the associated release of oxytocin cannot be underestimated. When it comes to pleasing your partner, your looks and your charming personality may not be the biggest turn-ons you have to offer. Your willingness to provide loving touch—even in those areas of the anatomy that aren't typically considered to be sexy—may be your greatest asset. In response to your gift of loving or sensual touch, your lover will undergo an oxytocin-induced emotional transformation. In the presence of oxytocin, bonding is facilitated, and your lover will experience a powerful rush of extremely positive feelings toward you, a distinct biological event that serves to strengthen your relationship each and every time it happens.

Engaging in nonsexual touching with your lover on a regular basis not only builds intimacy, but it also creates sexual tension and serves as an extended form of foreplay. When the time is right for lovemaking, the oxytocin-primed brains and bodies of both partners will be ready and willing for sexual contact. Mutual touching is vital to love relationships, and most of us don't give or receive enough of it to keep the bonds of intimacy as strong and as healthy as they could be.

Although touch provides a powerful stimulus for the release of oxytocin, physical contact is not required for its release. Visual and verbal cues, and even simple thoughts, can trigger an oxytocin surge. Many nursing mothers experience "letdown" of their breast milk simply by seeing an infant or hearing it cry. Sometimes, just *thinking* about their babies can initiate the secretion of breast milk. In studies of happily married women, researchers found that when they asked their subjects to think about their husbands, their oxytocin levels rose. Women in happy love relationships were found to have greater spikes in oxytocin levels in response to positive emotions.

Humans aren't the only ones sensitive to the sex- and relationship-enhancing effects of oxytocin. For years, researchers at Emory University have studied love behaviors using mouse-like rodents, called voles, as their scientific models. The research has focused on two particular species: the prairie vole and the montane vole. The two rodents are 99 percent identical in terms of their genetics, but in terms of their love relationships, the tiny genetic discrepancy between them makes a huge difference. Their radically different approaches to love and sex are most likely due to the fact that prairie voles are able to manufacture oxytocin, while montane voles are not.

Field biologists observing voles in the wild have documented stark contrasts in the social behaviors of the prairie and montane voles. Prairie voles are committed mates and lovers. Once a male and female pair up, they tend to spend most of their time together, preferring them almost to the exclusion of all their other vole acquaintances. When one of the pair dies, the other grieves its love loss long and hard, often to the point that it never attempts to seek out a replacement partner.

By contrast, the montane voles are loners. They breed promiscuously, and romance is little more than a slam-bam type of affair. While the devoted prairie vole couples typically spend more than 50 percent of their time cuddling, montane voles spend less than 5 percent of their time in close contact with another individual. Prairie voles are virtual fortresses of family values. Both moms and dads are affectionate, nurturing parents, and they provide lots of paws-on parenting to their cherished offspring. Montane mothers, on the other hand, offer little more than the barest of maternal essentials, and the deadbeat dads are usually completely missing in action.

In terms of human sexuality, oxytocin facilitates bonding and intimacy between lovers. But it also has more direct effects on sexuality. Higher levels of oxytocin result in greater sexual receptivity. Because oxytocin is known to drive testosterone production, it boosts libido in men and women. Oxytocin increases the sensitivity of the genitals and breasts, improves erections in men and sexual arousal in women, and makes orgasm more intense. And while oxytocin prods us to want sex, sexual activity increases the production of oxytocin. Stimulation of the nipples and genitals in men and women increases levels of oxytocin in the bloodstream. Orgasm causes the neurotransmitter to spike to levels that are three to five times greater than baseline levels, creating the afterglow of closeness that most people experience after making love.

Sexual activity increases oxytocin levels, leaving lovers in great anticipation of the next encounter. Oxytocin increases production of testosterone and estrogen, boosting libido over the long haul. Because of the oxytocin-sex feedback loop, its relatively safe to say that the more sex you have, the more you'll want.

SEROTONIN

In the human brain, the neurotransmitter serotonin can be thought of as the opposing force of dopamine. While dopamine fires off a chain reaction that leads to feelings of intense pleasure, excitement, and even euphoria, serotonin bathes the brain with a soothing sense of calm, relaxation, and in higher amounts, sleep. Dopamine is released in a pulsatile manner in response to certain types of stimulation, and its effects are immediately felt by way of a high-energy buzz. Serotonin, on the other hand, works at a much slower and steadier pace. In contrast to the sharp peaks and drop-offs seen with dopamine, serotonin tends to rise in gentle swells before leveling back off.

Although the actions of serotonin often oppose those of dopamine, each plays a critical role in human sexuality. In different ways, and in differing degrees of intensity, both neurotransmitters create feelings of pleasure. Serotonin can be thought of as a sexual moderator, serving as a set of brakes for dopamine's lead-footed sexual accelerator. It acts to smooth off the rough edges of sexual aggression that are triggered by dopamine. At the same time, it promotes a state of sexual readiness by calming emotional tension and alleviating anxiety, both of which can dampen sexual desire and make it impossible to relax sufficiently to enjoy lovemaking. Serotonin allows us to be receptive to the positive emotions that come with sexual activity, thereby promoting intimacy. Under the moderating influence of serotonin, we are better able to create and maintain selective and enduring sexual relationships.

In the absence of adequate levels of serotonin, sexual behaviors can become quite impulsive and aggressive. In one laboratory study, mice that were rendered serotonin-deficient began to exhibit promiscuous behaviors that quickly led to a kind of sexual free-for-all. They became indiscriminate in their choice of partners, mounting both males and females, and even animals of different species.

Obviously, some serotonin is necessary for appropriate sexual function. Having too little serotonin would make it exceedingly difficult to find a partner willing to tolerate your aggressive sexual behaviors. On the other hand, serotonin levels that are too high can be just as troublesome. This phenomenon is especially evident in individuals taking antidepressants belonging to the class of drugs known as selective serotonin reuptake inhibitors. These antidepressants work by preventing the normal breakdown of serotonin in the brain. As serotonin levels climb in response to the medication, depressed individuals start to feel better. They're happier, calmer, and more optimistic. But as their serotonin levels continue to rise, they may find themselves calm to the point of being apathetic. They may lack the initiative to seek pleasurable activities, and in the process, lose touch with their libido, and become totally indifferent to sex.

Serotonin and dopamine are known to share the same receptors in the brain. With serotonin molecules virtually saturating all the receptors, there's nowhere for dopamine to dock, even if it is released. As a result, high serotonin levels can result in the inability to achieve orgasm. As emotional flatliners, people with excessive serotonin aren't able to ride the exhilarating roller coaster of emotions that normally comes with sexual activity.

There's no easy laboratory test used to determine if elevated serotonin levels are at the root of libido problems or disorders of sexual arousal. Even if such a test existed, it probably wouldn't be all that helpful, since "normal" serotonin level undoubtedly varies from person to person. At the same time, anyone taking an SSRI antidepressant is certainly at risk for diminished libido and sexual response related to high serotonin levels. High-carbohydrate diets can also contribute to high serotonin levels. If you think that an imbalance of serotonin is negatively affecting your libido or other aspects of your sexuality, simply lowering the carbohydrate content of your diet and boosting your protein intake might be all that it takes to restore normalcy. If you're taking an antidepressant drug belonging to the SSRI class, a reduction in dose or a switch to another medication may be enormously beneficial to your sex life.

PHEROMONES

Unless you've ever witnessed a sow root for a truffle, you might not fully appreciate the power of pheromones. One tantalizing whiff of the truffle transforms what is normally a quite placid creature into a sex-crazed maniac. In her frenzy to get to the object of her fascination, she will dig, root, wallow in the earth, and assume provocative piggy poses, apparently oblivious to the amount of time, effort, or personal discomfort involved.

The truffle itself is not all that attractive, and probably not worthy of the sow's passion. It is, in fact, a rather homely root, perhaps even more so than the she-pig that lusts after it. Years ago, a German scientist, pondering the porcine fetish, set out to determine the reason for all the fuss. He discovered that truffles contain high concentrations of androstenol, a male sex hormone found in boars. Interestingly, the hormone found in truffles and boars is remarkably similar to sex steroids found in the human male. Although the effects of the hormone are certainly not as potent in people as they are in pigs, they still exist to an impressive degree. One study found that when women were placed in a room that had been sprayed with androstenol, they perceived men in photographs to be significantly more attractive than when the same pictures were viewed in untreated rooms.

The androstenol in truffles is a good example of a pheromone, a hormonal substance secreted by a variety of animals and insects throughout the wild kingdom. Creatures use pheromones as chemical messengers, designed to broadcast their sexual status and interests to potential mates. The male silkworm moth, for example, can pinpoint an eligible bachelorette almost seven miles away in response to a single molecule of her seductive signal.

With this in mind, animal pheromones and other animal products are used as ingredients in perfumes designed to attract members of the opposite sex. In its natural form, musk is derived from the male musk deer. A gland under the tail of the civet cat is the original source of the valuable fragrance civet, and amber was initially isolated from the intestines of whales. Jasmine contains small concentrations of skatole and indole, compounds that are normally present in feces.

In the not too distant past, it was commonly accepted that human beings were incapable of detecting or responding to pheromones—that somehow we had evolved past such primitive processes. A few upstart scientists challenged this dogma, and they've accumulated some pretty strong evidence to back their theory. One of the best known studies examining the effects of pheromones in people showed that women living together in group settings, particularly in college dormitories, tend to develop synchronized menstrual cycles. This study prompted others, and pheromones are finally beginning to get the respect they deserve.

The potency of pheromones was clearly demonstrated nearly forty years ago by now-famous scientist Dr. David Berliner at the University of Utah. While working on an experiment involving skin cells in his laboratory, he noticed that when the vials containing the skin samples were open to the air, the members of his staff underwent striking changes in behavior. Once subject to bouts of bickering, his fellow researchers displayed a new spirit of camaraderie and cohesiveness. When Berliner's experiment ended and the vials were sealed, his associates fell back into their old contentious ways. Upon reopening the vials, he again observed positive changes in their attitudes and behaviors.

After years of additional work, Berliner succeeded in isolating the mood-altering substances, and found them to be strikingly similar to those already known to stimulate sexual drive and activity in animals. Surprisingly, he discovered that while these substances are unquestionably capable of triggering behavioral changes in the people exposed to them, they are completely devoid of any scent. It became clear that because they were odorless, the substances had no effect on the human olfactory system, and thus, some other system was responsible for mediating their effects.

Berliner's conundrum eventually led him to pinpoint the organ responsible for this "sixth sense" of pheromone perception, the vomeronasal organ, or VNO. Although the VNO had been identified in humans decades earlier, it was commonly believed to be nonfunctional in human beings. In humans, the VNO sits nestled within the membranes covering the nasal septum. It has tiny, slit-like openings in each nostril. Berliner and his associates successfully proved that this organ acts as a receptor for a unique sensory system—one that is entirely separate from the sense of smell. To further establish that this "sixth sense" is alive and well in humans beings, they identified and mapped a pathway of nerves originating in the VNO and leading directly to the hypothalamus, the brain's control center for the most primitive of human emotions and drives, including sex, hunger, and fear. Messages derived from pheromones travel through nerves in the VNO that are parallel to—but completely separate from—the nerves in the olfactory system and deliver them to an entirely different part of the brain.

More recently, researchers at Rockefeller University in New York discovered what seems to be a pheromone receptor gene in the olfactory tissue of human beings. The gene, called V1RL1, appears to be fully functional, capable of receiving pheromonal signals from other humans, and then triggering emotional, biological, and physical changes in the recipient.

Several unrelated studies support the fact that a woman's sexuality is influenced to a large degree by her sense of smell, as well as by her "sixth sense" of pheromone perception. A group of Italian scientists demonstrated that women tend to have an exaggerated sense of smell immediately prior to ovulation, the period of time in which they are most fertile, and in many cases, most receptive to sexual activity. One study examined the effects of the birth control pill on the sense of smell in women. Sixty women, ranging in age from eighteen to forty were exposed to different smells at various stages during a single reproductive cycle. At the start of the study, none of the women were taking the Pill, and each was exposed to several different scents. The researchers found that the women's sense of smell was keenest during the time of ovulation, the period of impending fertility.

The researchers concluded that changes in a woman's sense of smell correspond to the fluctuations in her hormone level and fertility status and that this probably serves an evolutionary function. In response to scents and pheromones, a woman is driven to desire sexual activity at times in her menstrual cycle when she is most fertile and most likely to conceive.

The women were then asked to take the birth control pill for three months, and then they were again subjected to a round of scent-testing at distinct phases of their reproductive cycle. The same fluctuations were not observed. Under the influence of the birth control pill, the women's sense of smell remained constant, with no improvement noticed during the peri-ovulatory period of their cycles. Furthermore, the Pill-takers' sensitivity to smell closely resembled their level of sensitivity during the phase of their menstrual cycle when they were infertile and highly unlikely to conceive. It may not be a coincidence that this is also the period of time during which many women report low levels of sexual interest and diminished enjoyment in sexual activity. By suspending women in a state of unnatural infertility, the Pill may mask the effects of hormonal changes that boost libido. With this in mind, it isn't all that surprising that, of the women who stop taking birth control pills, nearly half cite the Pill's negative impact on sexual desire and enjoyment as a major reason.

Smell and pheromone perception may have a more important impact than just boosting libido and enhancing sexual enjoyment. Both senses may guide a woman to choose a mate who will allow her to produce strong, genetically sound offspring. Researchers at Sloan Kettering Cancer Institute in New York proposed this theory when they discovered that laboratory mice tend to choose mates that have significant differences in certain com-ponents of their immune systems. Proteins of the immune system, forming what is known as the major histocompatibility complex (MHC), are thought to be of supreme importance to mice—and other creatures—when it comes to selecting a mate.

The proteins of the MHC are present in nearly every cell in the body, in both mice and human beings. They are responsible for recognizing invading micro-organisms as not only foreign, but unwelcome. In the interest of pre-venting or overcoming infections and illness, they mobilize the body's immune system to destroy the offending agents. The proteins of the MHC are also involved in the phenomenon of rejecting organ transplants in human beings. Recognizing the donor organ as foreign, the MHC initiates its protective measures, which occasionally lead to the rejection of the organ, and the death of the organ recipient. Researchers at Sloan Kettering Cancer Institute found that the mice in their study were somehow able to detect key MHC differences in potential mates, and choose suitable mates accordingly. It is likely that pheromones are responsible for this phenomenon.

Apparently, human beings possess similar capabilities. In a study con-ducted at the University of Bern, women students were asked to smell the unwashed T-shirts of several different men that they had never met. When asked to rate the smells according to pleasantness, the women consistently favored the smells of men whose MHC were significantly dissimilar from their own. When researchers asked women who were currently taking the Pill to rank the shirt smells, those women preferred the smell of men with an MHC similar to their own. In light of these types of studies, women may be well advised to use some form of contraception other than the Pill when they're searching for potential partners.

Another study found that when women were given whiffs of several different T-shirts, one of which contained the scent of their own teenage son, they were most repelled by the aroma of their son's shirt. Researchers theorized that this phenomenon might have an evolutionary implication, preventing the disastrous genetic outcomes that result from inbreeding.

Male sexuality seems to be subject to the same factors. Although men may not be consciously aware that the women around them are ovulating, their bodies undergo predictable biochemical changes in the presence of fertile females. A group of Austrian researchers found that when men inhaled synthetic replications of women's vaginal secretions during ovulation, the men's testosterone levels increased dramatically. In contrast, men inhaling water vapor experienced a drop in testosterone levels.

Clearly, anyone interested in gaining the sexual interest of a potential partner would be wise to make use of pheromones and tap into the amazing sexual powers of the sixth sense. Although you can buy commercially produced pheromones, there's really no need to spend a dime of your hard-earned money on the synthetic stuff. You can find all the pheromones you need right under your nose—or under your arms, to be more exact. Pheromone production and secretion are dramatically facilitated by sweat glands in the skin, which are concentrated in the underarms and in the groin area.

Human beings possess two kinds of sweat glands: eccrine and apocrine. The eccrine glands are distributed throughout the skin on all parts of your body: They've been helping regulate your body temperature since birth. Their clear, watery, secretions are odorless, but packed with pheromones. Apocrine glands are clustered wherever you have hair—primarily around your groin and under your arms. These glands don't serve any temperature-regulating purpose, and they don't begin to function until puberty. Apocrine glands open directly into hair follicles, and hair provides a surface from which the secretions of the nearby eccrine glands emanate. Apocrine sweat glands are the main culprits in causing body odor, although their secretions aren't the real problem—they're sterile and they don't have an odor. Your skin-dwelling bacteria are really to blame. They feast on the oils released from the apocrine glands, breaking them down into rancid compounds and release noxious fumes.

With all that we know about pheromones, it is interesting to contemplate the rituals involved in modern-day dating. Both men and women typically scrub themselves squeaky clean, and then douse their bodies with synthetic perfumes and colognes. While these activities are designed to attract potential partners, they may actually have the opposite effect. Soap and water strip the skin of its natural oils and secretions, and any trace of a surviving pheromone that happens to survive is then masked with artificial scents. Robbed of their natural "smell prints," men and women may not be able to determine whether any chemistry exists between them. On date night, your best bet might be to shower several hours ahead of time, and then abstain from applying any artificial scents or smells to your body. By letting your own "smell print" shine, you're making use of the most powerful aphrodisiac known—your pheromones. When they waft into the nose of the right person, they might prove to be absolutely irresistible.

CHAPTER 10

THE SEX AND INTIMACY-ENHANCING LIFESTYLE

To a large extent, how well you live determines how well you love, at least in terms of sexual performance and enjoyment. Your body is your own personal sex machine, and it needs regular maintenance, exercise, and the high-test fuel that comes from a nutritious, balanced diet. Ultimately, your sexual well-being is built on the foundation of your healthy mind and body, and it is critical that you take care of both.

SLEEP

Sleep, like sex, is an area of life that modern Americans tend to neglect. Many of us seem to have little time for the luxury of sleep, and scant interest in the banal frivolity of sex. Maybe it isn't entirely coincidental that approximately half of American adults report feeling dissatisfied with their quality of sleep, and nearly the same percentage feel unfulfilled by their sexual relationships.

Sleeping has become almost a sin these days, joining the ranks of other modern-day quasi-crimes like smoking in public or failing to recycle your soda cans. If you're squandering your life away by sleeping more than five or six hours a night, you probably know better than to admit it. Most people consider the ability to survive without much sleep a quality that is both enviable and admirable—a sure sign that you're living an industrious, productive life in the fast lane. Overachievers who hustle along the straight and narrow path to success find that, after satisfying the almighty gods of career and parenthood, there's just not much time left for personal pleasure or self-indulgence.

Your body just won't buy it. In reality, sleep isn't merely a decadent luxury or a weakness of your mortal flesh: It is an absolute requirement of life, ranking right up there with food and water. In fact, you can function longer without eating or drinking than you can without sleeping. The mental and physical shutdown that occurs during high-quality shut-eye is necessary to allow your brain and your body a chance to perform essential maintenance and repairs. Just knowing that you need more sleep doesn't make getting it any easier. Over the past century, Americans have reduced their average total sleep time by more than two hours a night. Getting a good night's rest faces some fierce competition in a world that's open for business twenty-four/seven.

How much sleep do you really need? Everyone is different, and the amount of sleep needed to feel rested, restored, and able to function at maximum capacity varies from person to person. It even varies from genius to genius. Thomas Edison reportedly napped just about four hours each night, while Al Einstein required a full ten hours of sleep to feel rejuvenated. Even if you're not a card-carrying genius, you probably still need somewhere around eight or nine hours of slumber each night to remain fully alert throughout the day. In environments regulated only by natural light, minus sleep-thieving alarm clocks and light bulbs, most healthy adults will sleep for close to ten hours a night. No one knows for sure what determines individual sleep needs, but genetics and stage of life probably play important roles. Babies and toddlers require more sleep than adolescents, and the typical teen needs more sleep than a mature adult.

Several studies suggest that one-third to one-half of American adults routinely cheat themselves of the sleep they need. While some of us have trained ourselves to heroically fight the need for sleep, there's really no way to train your body to lower its pre-determined sleep quota. As a result, many adults are chronically sleep-deprived. Short-term sleep deprivation won't necessarily kill you, but regularly denying your body the sleep it needs can create some serious emotional and physical fallout. Sleep deprivation first affects your mood, leaving you cranky and irritable. As your sleep debt mounts, you may find that you have trouble concentrating, thinking clearly, and even staying alert. Short-term memory and decision-making abilities are shot, and reaction time and performance suffer. Ongoing sleep deprivation can lead to bizarre personality changes, including aggressiveness, paranoia, and hallucinations.

Denying yourself the sleep you need has similar effects to drinking too much alcohol. Like the intoxicated, sleep-deprived individuals usually don't realize the degree to which lack of sleep affects their moods, performance, or even their relationships. The mistakes they make range from minor mishaps to major disasters. Sleep deprivation was found to be a major factor in the Exxon Valdez mishap, as well as the Challenger shuttle explosion, and the nuclear accidents at Three Mile Island and Chernobyl. The U.S. Department of Transportation estimates that drowsiness is a factor in roughly two hundred thousand car crashes each year.

Making you more accident-prone isn't the only way that lack of sleep can harm you. Researchers at the University of Chicago Medical School recently studied the effects of sleep deprivation on healthy young men. They found that missing just a few hours of slumber each night dangerously altered their blood sugar metabolism, increasing their risk for developing diabetes. Sleep deprivation also increased the subjects' levels of cortisol, a stress hormone that, in high amounts, can foster the development of obesity and high blood pressure.

How do you know if you're short on sleep? If you're walking around like a zombie, that's your first clue. You'll know you're mildly sleep-deprived if you catch yourself dozing off during boring meetings or dull television programs. If you find yourself nodding off when you're behind the wheel of a moving vehicle, your problem is more serious. Fortunately, no matter how long you've been cheating your body of the sleep it needs, it doesn't take long to repay your sleep debt. Most people are able to overcome even long-term sleep deprivation by getting just two or three full nights' worth of sound sleep. If you've fallen behind, you'll definitely want to start hitting the sack a little earlier each evening. You might be surprised to find that when you're rested, your daytime productivity improves, saving you time in the long run. You'll undoubtedly be more pleasant, and better able to cope with life's endless stream of stressful circumstances. As your mood improves and your energy levels rise, you'll find that sleep has a wonderful rejuvenating effect on your relationships. Sleeping really isn't a sin—it's a necessity of life.

Insomnia

If you're lucky enough to fall into a deep and peaceful slumber the minute your head hits your pillow each night, you should count your blessings.

Millions of Americans aren't so fortunate. According to a recent National Sleep Foundation survey, over half of American adults report being plagued with insomnia at least several nights a month. Insomnia isn't a sleep disorder in its own right, but rather a symptom of another underlying condition. Insomnia is defined as difficulty falling asleep, awakening frequently during the night, or waking up too early and finding it hard—or even impossible— to get back to sleep.

This lack of sleep is taking its toll on the nation's pocketbook, to the tune of about thirteen billion dollars, the amount spent annually on sleep-inducing drugs and medical services. The indirect costs aren't as easily measured. Insomniacs by night are zombies by day—their job performance suffers, and they have higher rates of absenteeism and accidents. Nodding off at the wheel ranks second only to drunk driving as a cause of U.S. car crashes.

Fatigue is the hallmark of insomnia, but its other symptoms are just as troublesome. Insomniacs have trouble thinking clearly, concentrating, and even remembering. Over the long haul, missed sleep can lead to depression and anxiety; discord in relationships; and diminished sexual desire and performance.

Not long ago, sleep scientists believed that your brain and body take a well-deserved rest while you snooze, but, in reality, the opposite is true. During slumber, your brain is busy firing up nerve networks and storing memories. Downtime is critical for routine body maintenance. While you sleep, your body circulates about 70 percent of your daily dose of human growth hormone, the natural anti-aging elixir responsible for repairing skin and rebuilding bone and muscle. Sleep is vital to a healthy immune system. Even moderate sleep deprivation dampens the body's production of disease-fighting immune cells, making insomniacs more susceptible to everything from minor infections like the common cold to major illnesses like cancer.

Insomnia has dozens of causes, but in most cases, stress and poor sleep habits are the real culprits. If you toss and turn at night, a few changes in your routine might be all it takes to send you drifting off to dreamland. You should start preparing yourself for sleep long before bedtime. It's a good idea to avoid caffeine, nicotine, and other stimulants late in the day—these substances interfere with your ability to relax and fall asleep. You should nix the nightcap as well. Although drinking alcohol initially produces drowsiness, even one drink can interrupt your sleep during the night, and can contribute to obstructive sleep apnea. Regular exercise burns up unspent energy and helps you sleep more soundly, but not if you schedule it too close to bedtime. Workouts should end at least three hours before you plan to hit the hay so that your body has a chance to unwind afterwards.

If you've ever engaged in the age-old bedtime battle with small children, you know the value of a good nighttime ritual. A warm bath, a light snack, and a regular bedtime go a long way toward signaling your brain that the day is done and its time for lights out. Your bedroom should remain a sacred chamber where sleep and sex are the main events. Don't desecrate it by making it a place to watch television, balance your checkbook, or fold the laundry. If you use your bedroom only for its designated purposes, you can actually train your brain to associate that room with sleep. Mr. Sandman is more likely to come calling if your sleeping quarters are dark, quiet, and comfortable. If your surroundings are noisy, use a fan or earplugs to muffle unwelcome interruptions.

If you find that you're still wide awake within a half-hour of going to bed, call a time-out. Drag yourself out of bed and into another room (remember, the bedroom is reserved for sleeping and sex) and occupy yourself with something that is not stimulating, like reading the owners' manual for your toaster oven. At all costs, resist the urge to shampoo the dog or organize your kitchen cabinets. Accomplishing great tasks during designated dozing time only serves to reward you for staying awake. When you feel sleepy, haul yourself back into bed, and try again. If you've revamped your routine and you're still not snoozing, it's time to get some help. Your doctor will want to look for the cause of your insomnia and may prescribe medicines to help you rest in the meantime. Some medical conditions can significantly alter the quality and quantity of your sleep. Depression, anxiety, heart and lung disease, as well as the drugs used to treat these conditions all can have profound negative influences on sleep. The hormonal fluctuations that occur with menopause and andropause can significantly alter the nature and soundness of your sleep. Before dismissing sleep problems as being all in your head, a visit to your doctor for a complete checkup might be in order.

The good news is that most cases of insomnia are short-lived and temporary, and you'll eventually regain your ability to sleep soundly. Before you know it, you'll be counting your blessings, instead of counting sheep.

Naps

Naps are okay for cats and babies, but how about for grownups? As mature adults, most of us feel guilty about indulging in any form of daytime dozing. Nodding off unexpectedly can cause problems, but a scheduled nap can be enormously beneficial. If you don't get enough Z's on a particular night, a planned power nap the next day is a great way to recover from sleep loss. Swedish researchers studying the effects of napping on daytime mental alertness measured the alertness of volunteers at three different times—after a full night's sleep; after four hours of sleep and a short nap; and after four hours sleep with no nap. The people who slept four hours with no nap scored the lowest on alertness tasks, but those who slept four hours and then napped scored just as well those who got a full night's sleep. Mood, memory, and reaction time also improve dramatically after a short daytime doze.

Before you start to nod off, there are a simple few rules for successful napping. In order for your nap to leave you refreshed and recharged, it should last no more than twenty minutes. If you nap longer, you could wake up feeling sleepier and groggier than you did before you dozed off. There's a good reason for this paradoxical phenomenon. Your normal nighttime sleep is made up of about five ninety-minute naps. During these ninety-minute cycles, the first fifteen to twenty minutes are spent plunging into the stage of deep sleep. After about forty-five to fifty minutes of deep sleep, you come up for ten or fifteen minutes of lighter sleep. Your eyes dart around during this period of sleep, accounting for its name, "rapid eye movement" or REM sleep. Dreaming occurs during REM sleep. Because it's a lighter stage of slumber, you can easily be aroused from it. If all is quiet and you're not awakened, you plunge back down into deep sleep again and repeat the cycle.

When you take a nap, your body doesn't know that your sleep will be short and sweet. It simply enters your normal ninety-minute sleep cycle. If you try to sleep for forty-five minutes, your nap will end smack in the middle of deep sleep, and you'll wake up feeling groggy. You may even feel more tired and less alert than you did before. If you nap for twenty minutes or less, you don't give yourself a chance to plunge into deep sleep. As a result, you'll snooze lightly, and wake up feeling refreshed, restored, and rejuvenated.

If you want to time your nap for peak alertness, plan to wake up at least thirty to forty-five minutes before you need to be mentally sharp. Not only will this give you time to iron the wrinkles out of your face and get rid of that bed-head hairdo, it will also give your brain a chance to warm up. The best time for napping is in early or mid-afternoon, when there's a natural dip in your energy level. At this time of day, your biological rhythms are gearing down, lowering your metabolic rate and your body temperature. It's the perfect time for an afternoon siesta.

STRESS

More than 80 percent of American adults admit to feeling "significantly stressed" at least some of the time. Although stressors vary from person to person, their effects produce similar outcomes. Whenever humans encounter what they perceive to be a stressful situation, the age-old fight-or-flight response is activated. This response triggers the release of a cocktail of potent hormones into the bloodstream, primarily adrenaline and noradrenaline. In the short term, your body's reaction to stress isn't always such a bad thing. Spurred into action, your built-in responses can save your life in times of real danger by quickening your reaction time and giving you the razor-sharp edge you need to perform your best in challenging situations.

What is helpful in the short term is actually quite damaging in the long run. Over time, the effects of stress hormones on the human body are usually much more devastating than the potential threat represented by the initiating stressor. Chronic stress can lead to hypertension, heart disease, stomach ulcers, headaches, and a weakened immune system, not to mention depression, anxiety, and insomnia. All can have significant negative impacts on libido, sexual performance, and sleep.

Back in the old days (I'm talking about millennia ago), the stress encountered by our ancestors was physical. There were man-eating tigers from which to flee and territorial cavemen to fight. The human body was designed to respond with lightening speed to this type of stress. During the last million years or so, our environment has changed dramatically. Modern stress is almost always emotional or mental stress. In your lifetime, you'll probably never have to fend off a hungry predator or a testy caveman, but you will encounter financial crunches, looming deadlines, and interpersonal conflicts on a daily basis.

Although our environment has changed, the human body has remained steadfastly the same, and it seems that Fred and Wilma Flintstone just weren't engineered to live in a George Jetson world. The threats that caused our ancestors stress could—and often did—kill them. It paid to have bodies that responded immediately and dramatically to stress. Now, it's not the things causing us stress that kill us—it's our body's reaction to the stress. The physiological response to stress is pretty much the same whether you're facing a life-threatening situation or a minor hassle.

When the boss makes unreasonable demands or the Xerox machine malfunctions at work, you feel stressed out. It's highly unlikely that you'll be forced to engage your boss in mortal combat or flee for your life from the copier, but your body doesn't know that. It only knows that you've encountered a stressful situation, and, in response, it activates the fight-or-flight reaction. In a single moment, dozens of changes occur in your body, all with the sole purpose of keeping you alive. Powerful hormones are released into your bloodstream, preparing your body to spring into action. These "stress hormones," including cortisol and adrenaline, drive up your blood pressure, heart rate, and respiratory rate so that more blood and oxygen can be delivered to your working muscles.

Fat, cholesterol, and sugar are hastily dumped into your bloodstream to provide a readily available and easily accessible energy supply. Blood is shunted away from digestive organs and other body tissues and rerouted to muscles. The body is preparing you—at the most primitive level—to respond to the stressor by fighting, or taking flight. Your muscles tense. In anticipation of battle wounds, blood clotting is enhanced, and powerful chemicals called endorphins are produced to reduce your sensitivity to pain. All of these responses are helpful if you're going to duel to the death or head for the hills to save yourself from the enemy. But what if the enemy is just your boss giving you an unreasonable assignment with an impossible deadline, or your spouse delivering a little bad news about your bank balance? Modern civility dictates that you remain outwardly calm while inwardly, your body is reacting with all the intensity it would if you faced a life-or-death situation.

The preparations that your body makes for fight-or-flight cause significant, irreversible damage to your body. When blood and oxygen are preferentially delivered to muscles, routine maintenance and repair of other tissues and body systems are neglected. Reduced blood flow to your head can give you a quick case of brain drain that makes it difficult to concentrate or even act rationally. Stress can make you forgetful. Chronic exposure to stress hormones accelerates degenerative changes in the brain that lead to memory loss. In a Swedish study, elderly subjects with low stress levels performed as well as younger subjects in memory tests, while those with high stress levels scored 50 percent lower. In people with chronic exposure to stress, memory loss may be permanent. This may be protective in some ways—at least you won't remember what it is that's stressing you out.

The rerouting of blood during the fight-or-flight response is great for working muscles, but it can wreak havoc in your digestive tract, causing nausea, stomach cramps, and ulcers. Under the influence of stress hormones, you may be treated to alternating bouts of constipation and diarrhea. Initially, stress hormones boost the protective powers of the immune system, but over time, they actually blunt the immune response. Your neglected immune system may be unable to muster an adequate defense against minor infections or major diseases. Several studies have found that people who endure chronic stress possess low levels of disease-fighting white blood cells, making them more susceptible to colds and other common infections. A study at Ohio State University found that in people with high stress levels, wounds took an average of nine days longer to heal than similar wounds in patients who were not so stressed.

Emotional stress is an important trigger for heart attacks. Stress hormones increase the speed and strength of the heart's pumping action, making it work twice as hard as it normally does, and setting the stage for dangerous rhythm disturbances. While blood-clotting factors are extremely useful if you find yourself in danger of bleeding to death, in the absence of a mortal wound, they can end up hurting you more than they help you. With the stepped-up clotting potential of your blood, you're more likely to suffer a heart attack. Repeated activation of the fight-or-flight response is thought to play a significant role in the deaths of more than one-hundred thousand Americans who die suddenly and unexpectedly each year from heart attacks. Stress also increases your chance of suffering a stroke. Prolonged exposure to stress can lead to thickening of the carotid arteries—blood vessels that deliver blood to the front part of the brain. Blockage and injury of these arteries are the primary cause of strokes. Studies have shown that men who are most bothered by stressful situations are significantly more likely to suffer strokes than those who have more carefree attitudes.

Even if stress doesn't kill you, it can still make you miserable. It can worsen a number of skin conditions, including acne, hives, and psoriasis. Long-term exposure to stress hormones robs your bones of calcium and other minerals, increasing your risk for osteoporosis and debilitating bone fractures. Tense muscles may help you spring into action, but if you're not going anywhere, they end up causing fatigue, neck pain, and tension headaches. Chronic stress is frequently at the root of sleep disorders and insomnia. Stress hormones are the ultimate "anti-sleep" chemicals, as they're designed to increase your mental vigilance and physical readiness. Ironically, while stress itself hinders sleep, its physical and emotional effects actually increase your body's sleep requirements.

Stress can have varying effects on body weight. While some people suffer loss of appetite and body wasting, others develop powerful cravings for salt, fat, and sugar. People who overeat in response to stress tend to deposit fat in their midsections, an important predictor of heart disease and diabetes. Chronic stress has been linked to the development of insulin resistance, a condition in which the body is unable to use insulin effectively to regulate blood sugar. Insulin resistance is a primary risk factor for the development of diabetes. Researchers at the University of Amsterdam found that stressed-out subjects were sixty percent more likely to have type two diabetes than their more mellow counterparts.

Most experts now agree that stress is linked to cancer. While there's no proof that stress causes cancer, there's plenty of evidence to support the notion that it influences the progression of the disease. Several studies have shown that emotional support not only enhances the well-being of cancer patients, it also prolongs their lives. In a study of women with terminal breast cancer, those who participated in support programs lived twice as long as those who did not.

Because of the myriad physical diseases and emotional disorders it creates, stress can be a real killer when it comes to your libido and your sex life.

It also damages your sexuality through another route. Stress hormones share the same precursor as sex hormones, and since self-preservation will always take precedence over sex, chronic stress results in lower levels of sex hormones and a reduction in sex drive. Stress has been shown to dramatically impair sexual performance, especially in terms of achieving physical arousal and orgasm. Recurrent bombardment of your blood vessels with fat, cholesterol, and sugar can lead to narrowing and hardening of arteries throughout the entire body, including the genitalia, leading to disorders of sexual arousal in women and erectile dysfunction in men. On a more immediate basis, the fatigue, irritability, and depressed moods caused by stress can totally deplete you of your sexual drive.

The physiological responses that ensured the survival of Fred and Wilma Flintstone now hasten the demise of George and Jane Jetson. What can you do to keep your survival mechanisms from killing you? It would be helpful if you could spring swiftly into action every time you felt stressed. Taking a couple of swings at your overly demanding boss or fleeing from your bearer-of-bad-news spouse would do your body a world of good, at least in the short run. In the long run, you might end up unemployed, imprisoned, or divorced, so it's best to find another way to deal with your stress.

Of all the stress-relieving techniques known, exercise is the most effective. Physical activity puts a damper on insulin levels, lowers blood pressure, and slows the heart rate. During vigorous exercise, your body secretes biochemicals called endorphins. These chemicals counteract the negative effects of stress hormones and have a soothing effect on your brain and your body. Exercise actually makes your stress hormones work for you, rather than against you. Even a fast-paced, twenty-minute walk helps protect you from the damaging effects of everyday stress. While you're at it, maybe you can invite the person who stresses you out to come along with you—you'll both feel better.

Combating Stress

In the pressure cooker that is modern life, you might not be able to eliminate stress or even avoid it, but you can protect yourself from its damaging effects. Learning to deal with stress effectively not only improves your health, it may save your life.

- Cut back on caffeine. Caffeine is a strong stimulant that actually generates a stress response on its own. Caffeine contributes to muscle tension, insomnia, and stomach upset, and it intensifies the negative effects of stress.
- Get moving. Aerobic exercise lessens the damaging effects of the stress response by putting the fight-or-flight reaction to good use. When it comes to relieving stress, a twenty-minute walk is more effective than most prescription drugs.
- Relax. While the stress response comes naturally, relaxing does not. With a little practice, you can learn to slow your heart rate, lower your blood pressure, and relax your muscles.
- Get some sleep. Sleep gives your body the downtime it needs to recover from the negative impact of stress. Stressed-out people usually suffer from fatigue, and fatigued people don't sleep well. This cycle is tough to break, but it's an important part of coping with stress.
- Take a timeout. Whether it's a weekend getaway, or a five-minute break, giving your body a chance to rest and relax goes a long way toward alleviating stress.
- Be jolly. Finding the humor in stressful situations is extremely therapeutic. Laughter helps dissipate stress hormones, releases tension, and reverses much of the damage caused by stress.

Laughter

Whoever said that laughter is the best medicine really knew what he was talking about. Laughter is good for your emotional and physical health, as well as your sexuality.

Most of us have been laughing since we were babies. Spontaneous laughter is seen in infants as early as five weeks of age; it's thought to be an evolutionary means of rewarding harried, overworked parents for taking care of their offspring and helping to ensure babies' survival. By the age of three, just about everything seems funny: The average child laughs some three hundred times a day. With age and experience, the realities of life tend to sober us up. By the time we're all grown up and weighed down with the worries of the world, we're laughing a measly fifteen times a day.

Not much is known about the physiological mechanisms of laughter. It's thought that about four-tenths of a second after we see the humor in something, a wave of negatively charged electricity sweeps over the entire outer surface of the brain. Electrical impulses set off a chain of chemical reactions, and endorphins and enkephalines are released. These opiate-like substances are the body's natural tranquilizers and painkillers. They produce feelings of pleasure and, occasionally, even a natural high. In response to laughter, neurotransmitters are reflexively and immediately released, including mood-elevating serotonin and norepinephrine.

The same process squelches the production of stress hormones normally secreted during the fight-or-flight response. Laughter gives a boost to the body's disease-fighting army, the immune system. A hearty laugh has been shown to activate cellular soldiers called T lymphocytes and natural killer cells. It increases the production of immunoglobulins that protect the body from viruses and other foreign invaders.

In his book, *Anatomy of an Illness*, Norman Cousins proposed the use of laughter as a healing tool. Suffering from a rare form of painful arthritis, Cousins found traditional medicines ineffective and decided to cure himself with daily doses of humor. He discovered that when he watched Marx brothers' films and episodes of *Candid Camera*, his gleeful laughter helped him sleep better and stay more comfortable with fewer pain pills.

Laughing is good exercise. A hearty laugh is a good workout for the diaphragm, the lungs, and the muscles of the abdomen, face, and chest. Laughing increases the blood's oxygen level, improves circulation, and gently tones the entire cardiovascular system. When the laughter subsides, heart rate and blood pressure drop to below normal levels, leaving the laugher profoundly relaxed. This physical state of relaxation can last up to forty-five minutes, and is undoubtedly beneficial in countering heart disease, high blood pressure, and depression. Studies have shown that laughter is just as effective at reducing stress as biofeedback training.

Laughter is a natural coping mechanism—a healthy alternative to a stress-relieving cigarette or martini. Laughing leads to a cleansing release of emotion, and it's a socially acceptable way to vent pent-up frustration, and blow off tension. The state of relaxation that follows a good knee-slapper re-energizes you and helps you find positive solutions to life's challenges. If you can't laugh, you're in serious trouble. Avoiding laughter robs you of your most powerful coping tool—your sense of humor. If your funny bone is broken and you can't quite manage a hearty laugh, a simple smile gives you some of the same benefits. Smiling doesn't seem to boost your immune system quite as well as laughing, but it can dramatically lift your spirits. In one study, researchers asked volunteers to say "e" over and over. The volunteers reported an inexplicable feeling of happiness afterwards; they didn't know it was simply because saying "e" made them take on smile-like expressions.

Smiling is fine, but laughter is infinitely better. Laughter improves not only your own mood, but also the moods of everyone around you. Making someone else laugh creates a sense of belonging, connection, and intimacy. It can immediately erase feelings of hostility, resentment, or anger. Laughter improves your popularity and social standing; people are magnetically drawn to those who laugh easily and who make us laugh. If you're looking for a stress-reducing, health-boosting, libido-lifting aphrodisiac, laughter is it.

ALCOHOL

When it comes to enhancing sexual performance, one drink is fine, but indulging in more is asking for big trouble. Alcohol is commonly thought of as an aphrodisiac, in large part because it tends to wash away social and sexual inhibitions. One drink can trigger a delightful surge of dopamine, which increases your receptivity to the joys of sexual activity, and possibly your ability to engage in it. But drinking more than one alcoholic beverage can actually stimulate the production of serotonin in the brain, which in higher amounts can impair sexuality. Whether excess serotonin comes as a result of taking a selective serotonin reuptake inhibitor (SSRI) antidepressant or drinking too much alcohol, the effects are similar. At higher than normal levels, the neurotransmitter can interfere with a man's ability to sustain an erection, and a woman's ability to achieve a physical state of arousal.

Over time, regular, indiscriminate use or abuse of alcohol can interfere with the production of testosterone by the testes and adrenal glands. By lowering levels of the mineral zinc, it allows more testosterone to be converted to estrogen, an effect that can further diminish sexual desire and performance. By damaging the liver, it causes estrogen levels to rise even more, and can lead to sustained erectile dysfunction in men, and sexual arousal disorder in women.

That said, it's still okay to drink in moderation. As long as you're not morally opposed, drinking small amounts of alcohol might actually be good for your health. In a 1997 report featured in *The New England Journal of Medicine*, researchers found that when done in moderation, drinking reduces death from all causes by as much as 20 percent. This study shored up previous findings suggesting that drinking alcohol in moderation lowers the risk of death due to heart disease.

Interest in alcohol as a benefactor for the heart was piqued after researchers began to study the so-called French paradox. The paradox refers to the fact that the French, who habitually consume foods loaded with saturated animal fats, enjoy very low rates of heart disease. Their penchant for wine was thought to be the explanation for this confusing phenomenon. Since that time, moderate alcohol consumption has been found to protect against heart disease in several ways. Not only does it prevent fat from clinging to artery walls, an action that helps prevent blockage of the blood vessels, but it also boosts levels of heart-friendly high-density lipoprotein (HDL) cholesterol. In addition, it seems to have an anticlotting effect on the blood, accounting for the reduced risk of stroke seen in moderate drinkers.

Although these findings are relatively new, some doctors have long recognized the benefits of an occasional cocktail or a glass of wine to improve appetite and digestion, and to help their patients unwind at the end of a hectic day. But you'll rarely hear a physician discuss the benefits of alcohol without uttering the word "moderation" at least once in the same breath. The concept of moderation seems to be a little problematic, as the definition can vary significantly depending on who's doing the defining. What seems like moderation to brothers in a college fraternity may seem more like excess to brothers in the Baptist faith.

In light of these types of discrepancies, the federal government has taken it upon itself to remove the guesswork from the matter. The U.S. dietary guidelines define "moderation" as one drink daily for women and two for men. Since men tend to weigh more, have less body fat, and metabolize alcohol more efficiently than women, two drinks for a man has about the same biological effect as one drink for a woman. Volume-wise, one drink translates to twelve ounces of beer, five ounces of wine, or one-and-a-half ounces of eighty-proof liquor.

While a drink or two a day may help keep the grim reaper at bay, any more serves as a formal invitation to the ghoulish one. Although heavy alcohol consumption is associated with a low risk of death from heart disease, it's probably because other diseases get there first. People who drink beyond the point of moderation have higher rates of death from cancers of the liver and throat, not to mention deaths caused by accidents. Even more than men, women need to carefully weigh the risks and benefits of alcohol consumption. Women who drink just one alcoholic beverage a day increase their risk of developing breast cancer by about 10 percent, and two drinks a day bumps the risk up to 25 percent.

In some cases, you're better off to forego the benefits of alcohol and opt for total abstinence. Most doctors advise pregnant women to refrain from drinking until after the blessed event. Alcohol should be considered totally off-limits for recovering alcoholics, and ditto for designated drivers. Since more than 100 prescription and over-the-counter medications are known to interact unfavorably with even small amounts of alcohol, people who take drugs of any sort should find out about potential interactions. Alcohol can deepen the sedating and libido-depleting effects of some drugs, including antihistamines and antidepressants. Other drugs can become toxic or completely ineffective when mixed with a drink. If you're taking several medications, your best bet is to stick with beverages of the nonalcoholic variety.

If you've made it this far as a teetotaler, there's probably no really good reason to start drinking now. But if you're a moderate consumer of alcohol, it won't hurt to drink an occasional toast or two to your health, and to your sexuality.

CAFFEINE

If you would rather wake up to Mr. Coffee than to your dearly beloved, you're probably hooked on caffeine. Scientists have officially proclaimed you an addict if you habitually consume more than 250 milligrams of caffeine a day, equivalent to two cups of coffee. If you're an addict, you're not alone. Caffeine is the most widely consumed drug—that's right, drug—in North America, rivaled only by nicotine and alcohol. Americans drink more coffee than any other people in the world. The upside to all this caffeine consumption is that coffee gets us moving every morning. Low to moderate doses (30 to 200 milligrams) boost energy, wakefulness, and even improve some aspects of physical and mental performance.

The downside is that caffeine is addictive. Missing a single regularly scheduled coffee break can send you into a well-defined withdrawal syndrome with symptoms like lethargy, irritability, and a killer headache. Caffeine is a fairly potent stimulant, and drinking it too close to bedtime may cost you a few Z's. A single cup of coffee boosts your metabolic rate and increases blood pressure, heart rate, and adrenaline levels. The paradoxical sense of relaxation you get with that first cup each morning results from the undoing of the early symptoms of withdrawal. Coffee seems like a necessity, but there's no recommended daily requirement for it, and it hasn't been recognized as an official food group. In fact, coffee interferes with the absorption of important nutrients in your diet.

Caffeine prevents your kidneys from reabsorbing calcium—it actually pulls calcium away from your bones and reroutes it to your toilet. If you want to replace the calcium wasted by a single cup of coffee, you'll need to add a half-cup of milk to each serving. Drinking coffee costs you iron, too. Compounds in coffee called polyphenols bind iron in the digestive tract and prevent its absorption. Drinking coffee around mealtime can reduce iron absorption from food by almost 40 percent.

The caffeine in coffee has been accused of far more serious offenses, including causing cancers of the breast, colon, and pancreas, but these reports appear to be groundless. There is, however, some hard evidence linking coffee to high cholesterol. Hardcore coffee drinkers can lower their cholesterol by as much as 13 percent just by giving up their java. Coffee is thought to play an important role in cardiovascular disease. Drinking three to four cups of coffee a day may bump your risk of heart attack to twice the average, and drinking more than five cups a day can drive your risk to nearly three times the average.

As far as your sexuality is concerned, a single cup of coffee or caffeine-containing beverage may give you more energy and stamina for sexual activity, thereby enhancing your performance and overall enjoyment. When athletes drink three or four cups of coffee about an hour before they compete, they can outlast caffeine-free competitors by up to twenty minutes. This affect on athletic performance is real—so real that the International Olympic Committee has classified caffeine as a "restricted drug." Competitors are allowed to use caffeine, as long as they don't overdo it.

The rest of us can benefit from a little moderation as well. Consuming too much caffeine on a regular basis leads to chronic overstimulation of the adrenal glands, flooding the body and brain with hormones normally produced in times of stress. These hormones are known to negatively impact libido and sexual performance.

If you're like most coffee addicts, you probably have no idea how much caffeine you consume on a daily basis. Cup for cup, brewed coffee is the richest source of caffeine. And remember, a cup means just that—a measuring cup—not that two-gallon plastic monstrosity you got for your last birthday. One cup of brewed coffee has 80 to 180 milligrams of caffeine, depending on how strong you make it. Instant coffee provides about 60 to 100 milligrams of caffeine, and tea has 25 to 75 milligrams per cup. The caffeine content of a twelve-ounce soda ranges from 30 to 60 milligrams, and even decaffeinated coffee isn't totally caffeine-free: Most brands have 1 to 5 milligrams of caffeine per cup.

If you need a calculator to determine your caffeine intake, there's no doubt you're hooked. As with other drugs, too much caffeine can be dangerous, but you'd have to drink about seventy-five cups of coffee at your next coffee break to sustain a lethal dose. If you're getting close, maybe it's time to think about cutting down.

CIGARETTE SMOKING

Cigarette smoking is the leading cause of preventable death and disability in the U.S. Each year, more than four hundred thousand people will lose their lives to cigarettes, and countless more will suffer serious, debilitating consequences. Smokers risk shortening their lives by an average of thirteen years, and dramatically increase their chances of developing lung cancer, heart disease, emphysema, and a few dozen other medical maladies.

The tobacco rolled into each cigarette contains thousands of chemicals, including at least twenty-eight identified cancer-causing compounds. Some of the most powerful carcinogens in tobacco are substances called nitrosamines. Federal regulations permit only miniscule amounts of these carcinogens to make their way into other consumer products, like beer and bacon, but some tobacco products contain concentrations that are more than forty thousand times greater.

Other less-than-desirable chemicals in tobacco include polonium 210, a compound that is also found in nuclear waste; formaldehyde, also used as an embalming fluid; arsenic, a metallic poison; and lead, a deadly nerve toxin. The tar content in tobacco is responsible for much of the damage caused by smoking. Tar is the sticky substance found on tobacco leaves, and it coats and fills the tiny air sacs in the lungs. Smoking one pack of cigarettes a day for a year typically results in the accumulation of eight ounces of tar in the lungs, dramatically reducing smokers' ability to absorb life-sustaining oxygen from inhaled air. Insufficient oxygen in the muscle tissues contributes to fatigue and weakness, leaving many smokers too tuckered out to engage in sexual activity.

It's the nicotine in tobacco that keeps smokers coming back for more. Nicotine is one of the most addictive substances known to man, and, once you develop an addiction to it, overcoming it is incredibly difficult. Nicotine works through the same pathways in the brain as other drugs of addiction, including heroin and cocaine. All of these substances stimulate the release of dopamine, a neurotransmitter that produces intense feelings of pleasure.

Although the amount of nicotine in just one pack of cigarettes is a lethal dose, most people don't get enough of the toxin to kill themselves in the short run. The 8 milligram dose of nicotine found in a single cigarette is considered to be nonlethal, but that doesn't mean it can't kill you in the long run. Smoking just one cigarette elevates your blood pressure and revs up your heart rate, putting a significant strain on your heart. The effects of nicotine are evident within three seconds of lighting up. For the next ninety minutes, blood vessels in all parts of your body constrict, reducing blood flow to important destinations, including your heart, brain, and genitalia.

Nicotine contributes to the development of high cholesterol levels and hardening of the arteries. It also boosts your chances of getting blood clots, further increasing your risk for heart attack, stroke, and sexual dysfunction. Cigarette smoking is a significant risk factor for erectile dysfunction in men and disorders of sexual arousal in women. While cigarette smoking undoubtedly impairs your sexual performance, it may also make you look and feel less attractive. Smoking causes bad breath, stained teeth, receding gums, wrinkled skin, and accelerated graying of the hair. If you can't seem to quit smoking to save your health or your life, maybe you'll do it to save your sexuality.

Smoking Cessation

If you're like most of the nation's fifty million cigarette smokers, you'd probably really like to quit smoking, but quitting requires more than just wishful thinking. Because the addiction to nicotine is so powerful, you can expect your body to rebel when it is denied the drug to which it's grown accustomed. Hallmark symptoms of nicotine withdrawal include irritability, restlessness, difficulty concentrating, and, of course, a powerful yearning for tobacco.

If you're serious about quitting, there's never been a better time than right now. Before the era of nicotine replacement products, quitting smoking called for an iron will and nerves of steel. These days, dozens of products are available to help eliminate the physical symptoms of withdrawal, making kicking the habit easier than ever before.

Nicotine chewing gum, originally available only by prescription, has been offered over the counter in the U.S. since 1984. You're supposed to chew the gum slowly whenever the craving for a cigarette arises, so that the nicotine can be absorbed by the mucous membranes of your mouth. When used properly, the gum produces nicotine levels that are sufficient to stave off withdrawal symptoms. Common side effects of the gum include nausea, hiccups, and aching jaw muscles, but these tend to fade within the first week or so.

The nicotine patch has been available as an over-the-counter aid to stop smoking since 1995. The patches are easy to use—you just slap one on your skin every day and leave it there for eighteen to twenty-four hours. Aside from occasional, mild skin irritation, they seem to be well tolerated by most users. Nicotine inhalers and nasal sprays deliver the drug to your body via the mucous membranes of your mouth and nasal passageways. Although these devices release nicotine much more rapidly than the gums or patches, they may be less effective in the long run. Some experts believe that the rapid nicotine delivery actually reinforces addictive behaviors, making it harder to break the habit. Common side effects of nicotine inhalers and nasal sprays include irritation of the nose and throat, sneezing, coughing, and watery eyes.

Although all of the nicotine replacement products can be helpful, there's a much more powerful weapon in the anti-smoking arsenal. One of the most successful smoking cessation products is a prescription antidepressant medication called bupropion. Originally marketed as Wellbutrin, bupropion had the surprising side effect of contributing to spontaneous smoking cessation. This benefit was noticed in a study of veterans who were taking the drug for the treatment of depression. Additional research confirmed bupropion's effectiveness in promoting smoking cessation. This prompted the drug's manufacturers to seek FDA approval for its use as an aid to stop smoking.

Bupropion is now marketed under two names: Wellbutrin for the treatment of depression, and Zyban as an aid to smoking cessation. The most commonly reported side effects of bupropion are insomnia, headaches, dizziness, and constipation. Unlike many other antidepressant drugs, Wellbutrin is known for its relative lack of sexual side effects.

Although bupropion and the over-the-counter nicotine replacement products can help, becoming an ex-smoker still isn't an easy process. Of the twenty million smokers who try to kick the habit every year, only 6 percent succeed over the long haul. But even failed efforts are valuable—the average ex-smoker has logged five unsuccessful attempts before kicking the habit for good. If you want to boost your chances of success, you might want to consider enrolling in a stop-smoking program. Participation in support groups and formal counseling sessions nearly doubles the success rate achieved with smoking cessation products. Cigarette smoking is more than just a nasty habit—it's a dangerous indulgence that represents a tremendous threat to your health, your sexuality, and even your life.

HOLD THE SALT

If your idea of blessing your food is pouring salt on it, you're not alone.

Americans love salt, and each of us consumes an average of fifteen pounds of the stuff each year. Although you may crave salt, it's probably not a sign that your body needs it. As an adult, your appetite for salt is determined by deeply entrenched dietary habits, and has little relationship to your actual requirement for it.

Newborn babies have a natural aversion to the taste of salt—they grimace fiercely when they're offered salty foods for the first time. Until recently, salt was added liberally to baby foods—not for the baby, but to help get it past the official taste tester, the baby's mother. Faced with eating salt or starving, infants learn to tolerate it, and eventually even demand it. By the time these babies become adolescents, most will preferentially consume a diet that is incredibly rich in salt, featuring staples like pizza, potato chips, burgers, and fries.

Table salt is a chemical composed of two minerals: sodium (40 percent) and chloride (60 percent). In the body, sodium helps maintain the proper balance of water. The kidneys, in turn, are largely responsible for regulating sodium. When you eat a bag of potato chips, you create a sodium surplus in your body, and your kidneys dump the excess into your urine. When you mow the lawn in the blazing sun and lose a few pints of salty sweat, you create a sodium shortage, and your kidneys recycle it from your urine and pump it back into your blood.

In most people, this system usually works glitch-free their entire lives. But in some, the overworked kidneys may wear out and begin to have trouble getting rid of the excess sodium. The retained sodium holds water, increasing the volume of blood in the blood vessels and driving up blood pressure, leading to hypertension.

Hypertension is a serious problem in the United States, now known to affect about a quarter of the nation's population. Few experts claim that salt alone is to blame—of the millions of Americans with high blood pressure, only about 20 percent are salt–sensitive, reacting to excess dietary salt with a rise in blood pressure.

High blood pressure isn't the only problem associated with excess salt consumption. Weight gain and other symptoms of the dreaded premenstrual syndrome (PMS) are the likely result of sodium retention around the time of a woman's menstrual period. Extra salt leads to swelling of various body tissues, like those in the pelvis, causing bloating and pain. Swelling of the tissues around the brain can lead to headaches, irritability, and the infamous mood swings of PMS. Why premenstrual women crave the very substance that invokes such misery is a mystery— it's probably somehow related to Eve and the original sin. But giving into cravings for salt isn't wise—many doctors advise their PMS-suffering patients to stick to a low-salt diet the week before their periods.

By now, most Americans know that too much salt isn't healthy, but we can't seem to shake the habit. In spite of new low-sodium products and revealing nutrition labels, our consumption of salt hasn't changed much over the last century. Healthy adults require less than 500 milligrams of sodium each day, the amount in a quarter teaspoon of salt. Current dietary recommendations are rather lenient—we're advised to limit our sodium intake to 2400 milligrams a day. But the average American indulges in a whopping 7000 milligrams each day, the amount in three-and-a-half teaspoons of salt, and about fourteen times more than the body really needs or wants.

Where do you get all this sodium? About a third of it is poured from your saltshaker by your hand directly onto your food. The remaining two-thirds of it sneaks into your diet without a formal invitation: processed foods and fast foods are laden with hidden sodium. Since about half of the typical

American diet comes from processed foods, cutting down on sodium calls for some serious dietary changes. Not salting your food—especially before you've even laid your lips on it—is a good place to start. Reading nutrition labels can help you identify the big offenders. Most canned soups have over 1,000 milligrams of sodium, and a cup of sauerkraut has over 1,500 milligrams. A deluxe burger and an order of fries from your favorite fast food joint may contain well over 2,000 milligrams of sodium, allowing you to meet or exceed your entire daily recommended allowance in one sitting.

While switching to a salt substitute may seem like a good way to cut down on sodium, it's not advisable for everyone, and you should ask your doctor before you try it. Sprinkling seasonings other than salt is probably the best way to enhance the taste of food. It usually takes about a month or two to adjust to a low-salt diet and learn to like it, but if you stick with it, you can shake the salt habit for good.

CHAPTER 11

SEXUAL FITNESS

In the same time frame that Americans have experienced a serious lag in libido, exercise trends have tumbled along a similar downward spiral. While nearly half of Americans admit to having less-than-fulfilling sex lives, even more confess that they don't engage in any type of regular physical activity. According to the latest Surgeon General's Report on Physical Activity and Health, around 40 percent of the nation's population now lead totally sedentary lifestyles; another 40 percent engage in exercise only occasionally or rarely. It makes you wonder if the folks who aren't getting much in the way of physical activity are the same ones who report that they're missing something in terms of sexuality.

Although it is commonly overlooked, a close connection exists between regular exercise and a healthy, rewarding sex life. If you think about it, exercise and sexual activity are remarkably similar. Both can test the limits of your strength, stamina, and agility, and both leave you feeling profoundly relaxed, and even euphoric afterwards. Exercise and sex are also synergistic—any improvements in one area are likely to bring improvements in the other.

You don't have to be a world-class athlete to achieve sexual fulfillment, but it does make sense that the stronger you are and the greater your level of conditioning, the more easily you'll be able to meet the physical demands of lovemaking. Regular exercise dramatically expands your emotional and physical reserves, and with the boost in energy and vitality that comes with physical activity, going to bed doesn't necessarily mean going to sleep right away.

Physical activity enhances sexuality in several ways. For starters, exercise enhances blood flow to all parts of the body, including the genitalia. Not only does this action facilitate sexual arousal in women and erection in men, it also helps distribute sex hormones to target tissues throughout the body, especially the sexual organs. By improving your cardiovascular fitness, you'll be better able to withstand the rigors of prolonged and robust lovemaking.

By increasing your flexibility and tweaking the strength of the muscles throughout your body, you'll undoubtedly find that you can expand your repertoire of sexual positions. Toning and tightening the muscles of your pelvis will give you greater control over them, enabling you to accomplish the physically challenging feat of orgasm more frequently and more intensely. Possibly the greatest benefit of regular physical activity is the boost it gives to self-confidence and self-esteem, allowing you to fully embrace your sexuality and the myriad pleasures that it has to offer.

With all of the benefits that fitness brings to the boudoir, it makes you wonder why more Americans aren't taking advantage of the sex-boosting properties of regular exercise. Most people cite two reasons: They're too tired or too busy—or both. If you're too tired to exercise, that's a sure sign that you really need to get up and get moving. The energy you invest in exercise is immediately returned to you, with interest. Finding time to exercise is tough, especially if you have a hectic schedule and a life that seems full to overflowing. But the busier you are and the more stressed you feel, the more critical exercise is to your overall health and emotional well-being. Adding even a few minutes of exercise to your daily routine will undoubtedly pay off in terms of physical performance and mental acuity. You'll be able to tackle the day-to-day chores and challenges of your life with a little extra gusto. Increased efficiency and productivity in the short run will end up saving you a great deal of time in the long run.

Contrary to popular belief, you don't have to become a fitness fanatic or sacrifice huge chunks of your time at the altar of exercise to get all the blessings that physical activity has to offer. Even if you have just a few minutes a day to put your body in motion, you can reap the rewards of very real results.

In the not too distant past, fitness experts inadvertently dampened our enthusiasm for exercise by telling us that in order for physical activity to be beneficial, it had to be strenuous and continuous: at least thirty minutes a day, five days a week. We were led to believe that if exercise didn't leave us moaning, groaning, or having a near-death experience, it couldn't possibly be effective. Fortunately, this dogma has recently been ditched, thanks to some intriguing new research.

Several studies have demonstrated that for sedentary individuals who are currently overweight or out of shape, short, frequent bouts of activity are just as beneficial as longer, more intense exercise sessions. This notion is supported by the latest results from the Physicians' Health Study, a project that followed some twenty-two thousand U.S. male physicians for more than two decades. Data from the study reveal that men who exercise just eleven minutes a day are 35 percent less likely to suffer heart attacks than men who are total slugs. Interestingly, exercising for longer periods of time doesn't seem to lower the risk of experiencing a major coronary event by much more.

Men aren't the only ones who stand to benefit from brief, regular bouts of exercise. Several studies have demonstrated that women who walk just twenty to thirty minutes a day, either all at once or in ten-minute sessions, can achieve significant gains in strength and fitness, and lose weight at the same time. In light of these new findings, fitness authorities have begun to rethink their recommendations regarding exercise requirements. The American College of Sports Medicine recently revised its exercise guidelines, recommending that formerly sedentary adults strive to *accumulate* at least 120 minutes of moderate activity each week. The goal is to reduce the quarter-million deaths that occur annually in the U.S. that are attributable to a sedentary lifestyle: deaths caused by heart disease, cancer, and type two diabetes. As a bonus benefit, sexual performance and enjoyment improve.

No matter how hectic your life or how grueling your schedule, surely you can manage to squeeze in 120 minutes of exercise over the course of an entire week. If you do the math, it boils down to just about seventeen minutes a day. If you break it down even further, you'll find that you can get the exercise your body needs in two daily sessions that last just eight and a half minutes each. If you're already spending that much time watching TV each day, you can squeeze in a workout without revamping your entire life. You can jog on your treadmill while you're catching up on the news, or go through a simple weight routine while you're watching your favorite sitcom.

Even if you can't spare eight or nine consecutive minutes to devote to exercise, you still don't have to take a sledgehammer to your schedule. You can chisel away at your exercise quota a few minutes at a time. Try to squeeze in twenty sit-ups while your coffee is brewing each morning. Work in a two-minute workout by parking a little farther away from the office, and hoofing it across the parking lot. You can probably find a way to log a few minutes of stair climbing or brisk walking during your lunch break.

If you remember that doing any type of activity is better than doing nothing at all, and if you make fitness a priority, you'll be able to dream up dozens of creative ways to bump up your activity level in your life, just as it is. The idea is to get your body moving, at any pace, for any length of time. All you have to do is grab the opportunity to put your body in motion, and run with it, whenever you get the chance. If you can find just a few spare minutes in your hectic schedule, you've definitely got time to exercise. When you stick with it, the minutes—and the benefits—add up.

BODY IMAGE

If you look in the mirror and like what you see, congratulations. Your body image is healthy. On the other hand, if you find your reflection flawed, unattractive, or otherwise unsatisfactory, your body image could use a makeover. Whether it's good or bad, body image is the way you see yourself, and the feelings and beliefs you have about your physical appearance. Interestingly, it is often entirely different from the way others, including your partner, see you. What you think or believe about your own body isn't always based on facts, but rather on your feelings and emotions.

Regardless of their actual appearance, people with poor body image see themselves as ugly or undesirable and can't imagine that anyone else would admire their looks or find them sexually attractive. Their feelings toward their bodies can range from mild dissatisfaction to major disgust.

Having a poor body image can be emotionally and physically devastating. It can make sexual fulfillment impossible to attain. People who dislike their appearances are often guilty of failing to respect or nurture themselves, and they may even punish or neglect their bodies. Extreme dissatisfaction with physical appearance can lead to emotional problems, eating disorders, and withdrawal from sexual contact. Once a negative body image develops, it can take years to overcome.

A healthy body image is not something you're born with; it is learned. It is shaped by a multitude of factors, the most important of which seem to be family attitudes and the influence of the media. Children who grow up surrounded by people who value and accept them for who they are, rather than how they look, are generally satisfied with their bodies. But even with supportive family and friends, it's impossible to miss the "thin is beautiful" message delivered by the media. Television shows, movies, and magazines are dominated by lightweight men and women, and thinness is consistently associated with goodness, success, and sexiness. From the time we're old enough to notice, we're bombarded with images of ultra thin models who are anything but a true representation of real men and women. While our nation's population continues to grow heavier, our models are growing even thinner.

The gap between the ideal and the attainable is even wider today than it was just a quarter of a century ago. Back then, a typical female model weighed just 8 percent less than the average woman. Today's top models and so-called sex symbols weigh about 23 percent less than the average woman. Even professional beauties can't measure up to our society's rigid standards of perfection: Their photos are routinely enhanced via airbrushing and computer retouching. The unrealistic messages and images delivered by the media are largely responsible for making body dissatisfaction a prevalent problem in our society. The results of a 1997 survey published in *Psychology Today* revealed that 56 percent of women polled reported feeling dissatisfied with their overall appearance.

Although it is more socially acceptable for women to verbalize their dissatisfaction with their bodies, men are catching on and catching up. The *Psychology Today* survey revealed that 43 percent of modern-day men found their appearances to be unacceptable. Some experts believe that this upward trend is linked to the recent influx of men's fashion and fitness magazines, which has increased body awareness, and thus dissatisfaction, among men.

Not surprisingly, body image is closely tied to weight, especially in women. Nearly 90 percent of women and 60 percent of men surveyed said that they wanted to slim down. Achieving thinness was so important to them that 15 percent of women and 11 percent of men surveyed said they would be willing to give up more than five years of their lives in exchange for the ability to reach their goal weight.

Body image is closely linked to self-esteem and self-respect. When one is unhealthy, the others tend to suffer as well, and the end result is often unhappiness in many areas of life. Ultimately, having a poor body image can have devastating effects on careers, relationships, and sexuality. If you suffer from a negative body image, it's never too late to change. Learning to like and accept your body begins in your mind. You have to embrace the belief that ultimately it is your character and personality that make you who you really are, and not your looks.

On the other hand, if being overweight is the only thing standing between you and a healthy body image, you owe it to yourself to do something about it. Nothing improves self-esteem and self-confidence more dramatically than regular exercise.

Heidi's self-esteem and sexual self-confidence got a tremendous boost when she started exercising. "I wasn't terribly overweight, but I was getting really flabby. None of my clothes fit, and I couldn't stand to look at myself in the mirror. I definitely didn't enjoy sex—I didn't even want my husband to see me naked. All I could think about was how my thighs jiggled when I moved and how huge my rear end was." Heidi joined a gym and started a weight-lifting routine three days a week. "I definitely feel better, but more importantly, I feel better about myself. I'm proud of my body, and I want to show it off to my husband. When I look in the mirror and see sleek thighs and tight buns, I feel sexy."

One of the greatest kickbacks of exercise is the weight loss that comes along with it, especially in terms of body fat. Losing excess body fat is beneficial for a number of reasons: It helps normalize estrogen and testosterone levels, an effect that contributes to healthy libido and improves sexual performance and satisfaction. Losing body fat also lowers your risk of heart disease, hypertension, atherosclerosis, and type two diabetes. While all of these diseases reduce your quality of life and lower your life expectancy, they also dramatically increase your chances of suffering some type of sexual dysfunction.

Adults of normal weight typically have less than 30 percent body fat: Men have around 20 percent, and women have 28 percent. Lean, well-conditioned athletes, on the other hand, often have as little as 10 percent body fat, while obese individuals may be burdened with as much as 40 to 50 percent. While lowering your caloric intake through dieting can help reduce body fat to some degree, the best way to mobilize fat from its storage sites, bar none, is to engage in regular exercise.

During physical activity, stored fat is used to fuel working muscles. You don't have to run marathons or pump iron for hours on end; even moderate-intensity exercise is sufficient to trigger the release of fat from storage sites throughout the body. The more you exercise, the more efficient your muscles become at burning fat for energy. By increasing your muscle mass, you can transform your body into a calorie- and fat-burning blast furnace, and significantly lower your percentage of body fat and your weight in the process.

Exercise also fosters weight loss by promoting the release of appetite-suppressing neurotransmitters in the brain. With the increased energy that comes from regular physical activity, you'll be less likely to rely on food as a pick-me-up when you're feeling tired. Exercise revs up your metabolism—the rate at which your body burns calories. After engaging in physical activity, your metabolic rate remains elevated for hours, allowing you to burn more calories—even while you're resting—than you would if you hadn't exercised.

Several studies have found that when adults lose weight, they engage in sexual activity more frequently and derive greater enjoyment from it. Although improvements in self-esteem and sexual self-confidence undoubtedly play important roles, there's little doubt that there are physical factors at work. Sometimes, the pleasure derived from sexual activity boils down to simple mechanics—the ability to hold a certain position, or to support the weight of your body. By virtue of its bulk, excess fat deposits can make the act of lovemaking physically challenging. The extra work demanded of your heart and lungs to support your extra weight leaves less energy available to fuel your body during the exertion of sexual activity. As you lose weight and find new levels of energy, fitness, and stamina, you'll undoubtedly find yourself expressing your sexuality more freely, and enjoying it more.

When Regina, an elementary school teacher and mother of two small children, started exercising to lose weight, she gained a bonus benefit that she never even imagined possible. "Russ and I had basically stopped having sex. I was always too tired—I just didn't have the energy to make love." Regina had gained nearly fifty pounds during her last pregnancy, and by the time her youngest child went to kindergarten, she still hadn't managed to lose the excess weight. In desperation, she signed up for a beginners aerobics class at a local gym. "I was so out of shape that I couldn't even finish a thirty-minute session," she admitted. But she stuck with it, and within four months, she had lost nearly twenty-five pounds. Spurred on by pride and progress, she began working out with light weights twice a week at home. Within a year, she had lost just over sixty pounds. "I can't believe how much energy I have now! I can run circles around my kids. When I get home from work, I'm still looking for ways to burn off some of that extra energy, and a lot of times, I'll just attack Russ. I think we've made love more often in the past year than we did in the first five years of our marriage."

EXERCISE ENHANCES SEXUAL RESPONSE

One of the most important ways that exercise exerts its positive influence on sexual performance is by improving blood flow throughout the body. Exercise, like sex, increases heart rate, and, as a result, facilitates the flow of blood to the arms, legs, skin, and genitalia. Increased blood flow enhances sensitivity to loving touch, and reduces the likelihood of developing performance problems, including arousal disorders in women and erectile dysfunction in men.

The beneficial link of exercise-induced blood flow and sexual performance is documented in a growing body of scientific evidence. A recent Harvard study showed that men who exercised vigorously for twenty to thirty minutes a day were about half as likely to experience erectile dysfunction as men who were totally sedentary. A similar study conducted at the University of California found that when sedentary middle-aged men engaged in one-hour exercise sessions three to four times a week, they reported measurable improvements in sexuality. The former couch potatoes reported more reliable sexual functioning, more frequent sexual activity, more numerous and intense orgasms, and greater overall satisfaction with their sex lives. Most of the improvements are thought to be attributable to increased blood flow to the genital organs.

Shane is a good example of how exercise can improve sexual performance. When he came to my office over a year ago, he was forty pounds overweight and out of shape. His job as an air traffic controller kept him seated for most of the day, and he hadn't been involved in any type of regular physical activity since he played basketball in high school more than thirty years ago. He reported having trouble maintaining an erection, and he was concerned that his testosterone level was low. A thorough physical exam and blood work revealed that although his cholesterol level was slightly elevated, his cardiac stress test was normal. His hormone profile was within normal limits as well. He decided to try a three-month trial of exercise before undergoing further testing for erectile dysfunction. When I saw him back in my office, he looked like a different person. He was happier and more self-confident. He had started walking an hour a day after work, and had lost fifteen pounds. Even better, he reported dramatic changes in his sexual performance. Not only was he able to achieve satisfactory erections, he had more energy and stamina, all of which contributed to a much more enjoyable and fulfilling sex life.

Women who exercise regularly experience many of the same sex-enhancing benefits. Researchers at Bentley College in Massachusetts recently determined that women in their forties who exercise regularly engage in lovemaking activities more often, and experience higher levels of enjoyment than sedentary women. There is strong evidence to suggest that the improved blood flow brought on by physical activity can actually "prime" a woman's body for the physiological state of sexual arousal. In studies performed at the University of Texas, Austin, women were asked to watch an erotic film and rate their levels of sexual arousal on two different occasions: at rest, and, later, after twenty minutes of aerobic exercise. While the women viewed the films, scientists measured blood flow to their genital regions. After exercising, women showed an enhanced response to the erotic messages delivered by the film. In terms of both emotional and physical changes, sexual arousal occurred more quickly and more intensely after the women's bodies were primed by aerobic activity.

EXERCISE AND MOOD

Although the physical mechanics of sex are important, the emotional processes involved cannot be ignored. Chronic stress, depression, and anxiety are responsible for robbing adults not only of their libido, but also of the enjoyment and fulfillment that comes from the act of lovemaking. Fortunately, exercise is a powerful stress reliever and mood elevator. The exercise-induced release of endorphins and of the neurotransmitters dopamine and norepinephrine contributes to a state of emotional well-being, lifts libido, and improves enjoyment and satisfaction derived from sexual activity.

The powerful effects of endorphins first came to public attention in connection with the discovery of the "runner's high," a profound sense of euphoria experienced by athletes during periods of intense aerobic exercise. This natural buzz is a direct result of the mood-elevating actions of endorphins on the brain. The feelings of elation and optimism tend to persist long after the exercise session has ended. Many elite athletes are so addicted to the endorphin rush that comes with intense exercise that they are almost compulsively driven to achieve it. There's a perfectly logical explanation for this phenomenon. Endorphins are chemically similar to morphine and heroin. They're so similar that they actually bind to the same receptors in the brain, and trigger many of the same responses in the brain and body. Like morphine and heroin, they can be powerfully addictive substances.

Physical activity also reverses many of the damaging consequences of the fight or flight response. Like sex, exercise allows you to forget about your endless "to do" list for at least a few minutes each day. A brief exercise escape gives you a little time to traipse around in your own head and be alone with your thoughts. The endorphins that are released during exercise counteract the negative effects of stress hormones, and have a soothing effect on your brain and your body. These biochemicals also help alleviate anxiety and depression, which helps explain the fact that regular exercisers are much less likely to suffer emotional and psychological disorders.

When I first saw Stan over three years ago in my office, it was obvious that he was at least a little depressed. His hair was in need of a trim; he slumped in his chair; and he seemed to have a hard time making eye contact. Six months previously, he had been promoted to the position of maintenance supervisor at his job in a paper mill, and he was having trouble adjusting to his new level of authority. "I just don't know if I'm cut out for this kind of work. I'm stressed out all the time, and it's affecting the rest of my life. I don't feel like doing anything. When I come home from work, I just sit on the couch and watch TV. I haven't felt like making love to my wife since I took this job."

Stan had struggled with minor depression in his twenties, after the death of his father. He had taken an antidepressant then, and he didn't want to try it again. "I don't know if it really helped that much—it just made me sleepy. It definitely interfered with my sex life, and that's the last thing I need right now." Stan allowed me to refer him to a counselor, and, reluctantly, he agreed to start exercising. When he canceled his follow up appointment a month later, I phoned him at home. He thanked me for calling, and said that his life—and his sexuality—were getting back to normal. The counseling was helping. "The exercise is the main thing. My wife and I started cycling again, and it's making a huge difference in my life. I had forgotten how much I love it, and how great it makes me feel. I think I can handle it from here."

Exercise isn't necessarily a cure for depression, but it definitely helps. Dozens of studies have shown that people who are regularly physically active have lower rates of anxiety and depression, and are better able to cope with stress. In people suffering from depression, exercise significantly improves treatment outcomes and enhances recovery.

EXERCISE THROUGHOUT THE AGES

No matter what your age, it's never too late to start exercising. In fact, the older you are, the more important it is to pay close attention to your activity level. In older adults, regular exercise has been proven to reduce the risk of illness, and even death. A recent Harvard study found that physical activity can increase life expectancy, even among people who don't start exercising until the age of seventy-five.

The changes that occur with aging make exercising more of a challenge. The most noticeable changes involve the musculoskeletal system. With time, joints lose their mobility, ligaments become less flexible, and muscle strength and endurance steadily decline. Lean muscle mass gradually dwindles away, while the percentage of body fat steadily increases. Muscle strength is normally well-maintained until the fifth decade of life. Most folks experience a 15 percent drop in muscle strength from the fifth to seventh decades, and up to a 30 percent drop per decade after the age of seventy. It's likely that these changes will affect all areas of your life, but they'll be most noticeable in terms of the limitations they impose on your sexual performance.

Although the changes may be less noticeable, aging also affects the cardiovascular system. Blood vessel walls harden, and the heart muscle grows thicker, resulting in high blood pressure, heart disease, and sexual dysfunction. The lungs become less elastic, and lose some of their ability to take in oxygen.

Exercise won't completely stop the hands of time, but it can help offset many of the changes that accompany aging. It can dramatically improve overall health, as well as muscle strength, endurance, and flexibility. Regular physical activity helps lower blood pressure and improves oxygen delivery throughout the body. It lowers the risk of heart disease by boosting levels of heart-protecting high-density lipoproteins, while reducing levels of harmful low-density lipoproteins. All of these actions can enhance sexual function and performance in addition to improving your overall health.

Another sex-enhancing aspect of exercise is its role in regulating hormonal levels in older men and women. Staying active throughout your life is an effective way to combat the natural decline in testosterone levels. Regular exercise has been shown to increase production of testosterone, an effect that can elevate libido in both men and women.

AEROBIC EXERCISE

Aerobic exercise is any activity that elevates your heart rate for a sustained period of time and improves the flow of blood to all parts of the body. Jogging, cycling, and swimming are good examples, but any activity that puts your body in motion for at least twenty minutes is likely to qualify. For the beginning fitness buff, walking is an incredibly effective form of aerobic exercise. It doesn't require any special training, equipment, or athletic expertise, and it's a relatively low-risk activity. It's also convenient—just slip into some comfy clothes and a pair of good walking shoes, and you're ready to go.

Like all types of aerobic activity, walking elevates your heart rate, while it tones and shapes your muscles. It burns calories and facilitates weight loss, both during the exercise and afterward. Walking just thirty minutes a day three times a week has been shown to reduce the risk of developing heart disease by almost 50 percent. As an aerobic exercise, walking strengthens the heart, lowers the chances of developing high cholesterol levels, high blood pressure, and type two diabetes. These illnesses are dangerous in and of themselves, but they're also known to be significant risk factors for the development of sexual dysfunction.

If you're looking for new ways to exercise aerobically, don't forget that sexual activity counts. Lovemaking elevates your heart rate and increases blood flow. It gives your muscles and your cardiovascular system an invigorating workout. Several studies have documented the link between an active sex life and longevity. Welch researchers recently confirmed that men and women who engage in regular, enjoyable lovemaking have a lower risk for heart attacks and strokes, even when their sexual activity isn't especially rigorous. An English study found that men who reported having at least three orgasms a week were half as likely to die from complications of heart disease as men who were less sexually active.

RESISTANCE TRAINING

Regardless of your age, gender, or current level of fitness, resistance training can be enormously beneficial to your physical, emotional, and sexual health. Working out with weights improves your health in several ways. It increases bone mineral density, reducing the risk of developing osteoporosis. It improves conditioning and helps control pain in folks with arthritis and chronic back problems. It helps prevent and control type two diabetes by improving blood sugar and insulin levels.

For people trying to slim down, pumping up can work wonders. Resistance training increases the percentage of muscle mass in the body. Muscle tissue is a metabolic inferno, while fat is metabolically comatose. Pound for pound, muscle burns nearly two to three times as many calories as fat. The more muscle you add to your body, the higher your metabolic rate, and the more calories you burn, even while you're at rest.

One of the most attractive features of weight training is that even modest efforts can produce very real results. You don't have to hit the gym for hours every day to make major gains and realize dramatic differences in your body. While most traditional weight-lifting programs involve working out three days a week, even two days a week of resistance training is incredibly effective. In the first few months of your exercise program, lifting weights just twice weekly is nearly 90 percent as effective as working out three times a week.

Pumping iron a couple of times each week won't put a huge dent in your overcrowded schedule. It also allows more time for muscle recuperation and dramatically increases the likelihood that you'll stick with the program.

For beginning weight lifters, resistance machines with adjustable weight stacks are generally recommended since they're safer and easier to use than free weights. Resistance machines allow you to start with an initial load that is light in weight, and work your way up in small increments. Weight machines are designed to protect your lower back, reducing the likelihood that you'll stress or strain the muscles of your spine. While barbells and dumbbells require you to balance and control the weights on your own, resistance machines don't, so you'll be less likely to sustain an injury.

Working out with weight machines requires less time than free weight exercises, allowing you to comfortably complete your entire routine in as little as half an hour. Since exercise programs lasting longer than an hour have high injury and dropout rates, lengthy workouts aren't recommended, especially when you're just getting started.

Weight lifting makes a huge difference in your appearance, strength, and sexuality. It has a tremendous impact on neurochemical and hormonal secretion throughout the body. Strength training can tone and condition just about every muscle in the body, including the muscles of the pelvis, which can lead to more pleasurable sex, as well as more frequent and more intense orgasms. The enhanced sense of body awareness that comes with weight training helps put you in touch with your sexuality and gives you the ability and the desire to expand your sexual horizons.

PELVIC EXERCISES

Pelvic exercises help tone the muscles used during sex and keep them flexible. Both actions facilitate orgasm. Since the stretching exercises themselves can be quite arousing, you may want to try these at home with your partner.

Pelvic Lift

Lie on your back with your knees bent and slightly apart. Your feet should be flat on the floor; arms relaxed at your sides. Inhaling, tighten the muscles of your abdomen and buttocks as you lift your pelvis off the floor. Make sure that your back is straight, and not arched. Try to keep your abdominal and buttock muscles contracted for at fifteen least seconds, and don't forget to breathe while you're at it. Exhale as you lower your pelvis back to the floor, and then repeat the exercise a couple of times. As your muscle strength improves, you can increase the number of repetitions and the length and strength of the contractions with each session.

Butterfly Stretch

Lying on your back, keep your knees bent with feet together, flat on the floor. Pull your feet in toward your buttocks, allowing your soles to touch. As you gradually allow your knees to fall outward, you'll feel a gentle stretch along your inner thighs. Try to hold this stretch for thirty seconds, and then bring your knees gently back together. You and your partner can also try this exercise together, sitting back to back with spines touching. Relax your shoulders, and keep your head in line with your spine. Bring your feet in as close to your body as is comfortable, turning them so that the soles of your feet touch each other and your knees point outward. Clasp your feet with your hands, and allow your knees to slowly lower toward the floor, gently stretching the muscles of your inner thighs.

CHAPTER 12

THE NEW SEX HORMONE DIET

YOUR SEXUAL HEALTH DEPENDS ON A NUMBER OF PHYSICAL AND EMOTIONAL factors related to your overall health. Proper function of the glands involved in the production of sex hormones ensures that your levels of estrogen and testosterone are optimal, enhancing libido and improving sexual performance. Good circulation is vital to ensure the delivery of the sex hormones to their appropriate target organs, namely the brain and genitalia. The physical state of sexual arousal, manifesting itself as engorgement in women and erection in men also depends on a healthy circulatory system. The heart and skeletal muscles must be strong enough to withstand the rigors of sexual activity. The production of a balanced mix of neurochemicals in the brain is essential for driving sexual desire and enhancing sexual pleasure.

All of these factors are profoundly influenced by the foods that you eat on a daily basis. Your body requires specific nutrients to produce sex hormones and to maintain the health and proper function of the glands that manufacture them. In the absence of certain essential nutrients, your brain may not be able to produce specific neurochemicals that are vital to your sexuality and emotional health. Diets that are rich in fat and high in cholesterol contribute to hardening of the arteries and poor circulation, conditions that are linked not only to heart disease, but to sexual dysfunction as well. If you're not including enough high-energy foods in your diet, you're likely to feel too weak to engage in sexual activity or to derive much pleasure from it when you do.

The best diet for optimum sexual health is one that promotes good health in general. These days, eating well can be confusing. At any given time, there are hundreds of diet books available, with dozens of different eating plans. Many of them offer conflicting and confusing advice. While some of these diet plans are basically nutritionally sound, others are nutritionally incomplete and can be disastrous to your long-term health.

If you're looking for an eating program that is as easy to follow as it is nutritionally complete, your best bet may be to get back to basics, which, in this case, means the five food groups recommended by the USDA Food Guide Pyramid. Health benefits of following the food guide pyramid have been documented in hundreds of studies conducted by the nation's top nutrition experts. Eating foods from the five basic food groups in the recommended proportions is an excellent way to help lower your risk of developing diabetes, high-cholesterol levels, obesity, heart disease, and sexual dysfunction.

The food guide pyramid contributes to good health by allowing you to choose from a wide variety of nutritious selections from the five major food groups, which consist of the following:
- Meat, poultry, fish, dry beans, eggs, and nuts
- Milk, yogurt, and cheese
- Fruits
- Vegetables
- Bread, rice, cereal, and pasta
- Fats, oils, and sweets, in moderation

With so many choices, it's easy to meet your body's daily nutrient requirements for essential vitamins, minerals, and fiber, as well as carbohydrates, proteins, and fats. When you follow the serving recommendations of the pyramid, you'll be getting these nutrients in a balance that optimizes your energy levels, and gives you the strength and vitality to engage in sexual activity. Because it's low in fat and cholesterol, you'll be less likely to suffer from sexual dysfunction as a result of blocked arteries and poor circulation. The rich supply of vitamins and minerals helps ensure the health and proper function of the glands that regulate hormone production. By choosing foods from each of the five food groups that are known to promote sexual health and boost libido, your diet will make an important contribution to your sexuality, and make it easier to enjoy all of the pleasures that it brings to your life.

BREAD, RICE, CEREAL, AND PASTA

Whole grain breads, cereals, rices, and pasta are good sources of fiber and essential B vitamins and minerals, all of which are important to your health and sexuality. They're also excellent sources of complex carbohydrates, which, in spite of the overwhelming popularity of low-carb diets, are not the dietary villains they've been portrayed as. Carbohydrates are actually an important part of a healthy diet.

As it turns out, there are two types of dietary carbohydrates: simple and complex. Both are made up of smaller building blocks, which are sugars. Simple carbohydrates, like those found in cookies, candy, and other junk foods, are the real bad guys. These are the types that are quickly and easily broken down into sugar in the digestive tract, and they tend to wreak havoc with blood sugar and energy levels. Including too many simple carbohydrates in your diet may contribute to the development of type two diabetes and obesity.

Complex carbohydrates, on the other hand, are the good guys. Because of their complex structure, they are more difficult to break apart in the digestive system, and the individual sugar molecules that comprise them are released into the bloodstream more slowly. Eating foods that are rich in complex carbohydrates curbs your appetite and keeps you energized for hours. Elite endurance athletes have known this for years: That's why they routinely engage in the practice of "carbohydrate loading" in preparation for rigorous training sessions and competitive events.

Not only do complex carbohydrates act as high-quality fuel for sexual activity, they also stimulate the body's production of serotonin and norepinephrine, two naturally occurring chemicals in the central nervous system that are important regulators of mood and sexual desire.

While foods comprised of simple carbohydrates—including chips, cookies, and white bread—should be eaten very sparingly, you should strive to include six to eleven servings of whole grain breads, pasta, or cereals in your daily diet. A serving size is the equivalent of one slice of bread, one cup of ready-to-eat cereal, or a half-cup of pasta, rice, and cooked cereals.

FIBER

Fiber forms the structural framework of plants, but human beings have found a better use for it in their diets, and not because it's especially nutritious. Human beings lack the necessary enzymes to digest fiber, so most of its calories, vitamins, and minerals stay locked inside. Fiber travels through your digestive tract basically undigested and unchanged, and that's what makes it so useful.

A high-fiber diet reduces blood cholesterol by at least two different mechanisms. Bacteria in your colon convert fiber to products that eventually block the formation of cholesterol. Fiber also binds with formed cholesterol, preventing it from being absorbed into your bloodstream. A high-fiber diet helps your body excrete cholesterol, as opposed to depositing it along the walls of your arteries. Lowering your cholesterol level not only decreases your risk of heart disease, it reduces the likelihood that you'll experience some type of sexual dysfunction.

High-fiber foods can help you lose weight. Fiber-rich foods are bulky, filling, and low in calories, and they require some serious chewing. Because they take longer to eat, they have a higher satiety value than low-fiber foods. Fiber pushes food through your gastrointestinal tract at a steady clip, allowing less time for calories to be absorbed into your bloodstream.

All fiber is good for you, but there are two different types, each with important health benefits. Water-soluble fiber is found in products like oat bran, whole-wheat products, and the skins of fruits and vegetables. If you want to lower your cholesterol level, water-soluble fiber is the type for you.

The current recommendation for fiber intake is twenty to thirty-five grams a day, with roughly equal amounts of soluble and insoluble fiber. That's a lot—most of us eat less than half that amount. You don't have to eat a bale of hay to get your fiber, but you probably can't get it all by eating fruits and veggies alone. It takes about five servings of fruits and vegetables and six servings of whole-grain, breads, cereals, and legumes every day to get the recommended amount.

A fiber-rich diet will definitely improve your health—as long as you don't get carried away. Eating more than fifty grams a day can actually be harmful to your sexual health. When it is eaten in excess, fiber binds to zinc and other minerals that are important to sexual function, carrying them out of the body via the digestive tract rather than allowing them to be absorbed into the bloodstream.

FRUITS AND VEGETABLES

Fruits and vegetables are an important part of your healthy diet for several reasons. For starters, they're loaded with vitamins and minerals that are critical to the proper function of the sex glands, as well as to the production and regulation of the sex hormones. With the notable exceptions of the coconut and the avocado, fruits and vegetables are basically fat-free and low in calories. They're also excellent sources of fiber.

In general, the darker the fruit or vegetable, the greater its vitamin and mineral content. Nutritionally speaking, dark green, leafy vegetables, like spinach and spring greens, are better for you than light greens, like iceberg lettuce. Richly colored red and purple grapes are more nutritious than their paler green counterparts.

FREE RADICALS

Although most of us like to compare the aging of our bodies to the aging of fine wine, some scientists are more likely to compare it to the rusting of an old car, or the decay of a piece of overripe fruit. One of the leading theories on how we age is the oxidation theory, proposed by scientists who claim that aging is basically a form of rusting. When iron is exposed to oxygen, iron oxide—also known as rust—forms. Vegetable matter, when exposed to oxygen, begins to rot. The human body undergoes a similar process of decay: It's an inevitable side effect of living in an atmosphere full of oxygen.

Oxygen seems innocent enough—it's vital for the performance of almost every body function, and even for life itself. But oxygen also permits the formation of potentially toxic compounds in the body called free radicals. Free radicals are extremely unstable molecules, bursting with excess energy. They try to stabilize themselves by transferring their energy to any available bystander. If the energy is transferred to a key cell, tissue, or gland, serious damage can result. The affected molecule could be rendered incapable of functioning normally, or it could be completely destroyed.

If these renegade free radicals find their way into the control center of the cell, they could scramble our precious genetic material, DNA. Some researchers believe that DNA receives about ten thousand free radical "hits" every day. If the injury isn't intercepted by our bodies' natural defenses, the DNA may be left unable to program cells to divide properly or repair themselves, triggering processes that can lead to abnormal cell growth and cancer.

While free radicals are best known for their proposed role in cancer, they've also been blamed for causing the formation of scar tissue throughout the body. This scar tissue replaces normal tissue, preventing it from fulfilling its normal function. Depending on its location, scar tissue is responsible for wrinkles, cataracts, Alzheimer's disease, and sexual dysfunction. In the bloodstream, free radicals promote the formation of cholesterol plaques that lead to heart attacks, strokes, and sexual arousal disorders. In the joints, they initiate the degenerative changes that lead to arthritis. Repeated free radical assaults ultimately lead to a breakdown of all body systems, and the cumulative result is the aging process.

Fortunately, human beings have internal mechanisms designed to protect them against the formation of dangerous free radicals. Our bodies naturally produce lifesaving compounds called antioxidants. These molecular scavengers deactivate free radicals before they're able to wreak havoc on cells and tissues. Antioxidants found naturally in the body include vitamin E and C, the mineral selenium, and an enzyme called superoxid dismutase (SOD). Animals with the longest life spans appear to have the highest levels of SOD—humans seem to have the most. These natural antioxidants restore stability to free radicals and prevent them from dangerously reacting with neighboring cells. In doing so, they slow or even stop the oxidation process, reducing the incidence of cancer, degenerative diseases, and sexual dysfunction.

As we age, our natural defenses weaken, leaving us more vulnerable to the oxidative damage of free radicals. One of the best ways to prevent excessive free radical formation is to avoid substances that promote their formation. Radiation, ultraviolet light, cigarette smoking, smog, and unhealthy types of dietary fat are all believed to trigger free radical production in the body. Scientists have proposed another way to reduce free radical formation. Eating foods that are rich in antioxidants may help reduce oxygen damage and slow the breakdown of cells and tissues. Antioxidant compounds have long been used as preservatives to retard the spoilage of food and as antirust compounds to prevent the corrosion of metal. In a similar manner, dietary antioxidants may slow the decay of the human body.

You don't have to spend a fortune at the health food store on antioxidant pills and supplements. To date, no antioxidant pill has been shown to be more beneficial than eating a well-balanced diet. The most effective antioxidants are those that come straight from the packages provided by nature—fresh fruits and vegetables.

While fruits and vegetables are rich sources of the vitamins and minerals that are important to sexual function, they can also lower your risk of most types of cancer. The American Cancer Society recommends eating at least five servings of fruits and vegetables each day—recent surveys indicate that only about 10 percent of Americans routinely consume this amount. Diets that are lacking in plant foods are estimated to account for nearly 80 percent of cancers of the breast, prostate, and bowel. Studies have shown that Americans with the lowest dietary intake of fruits and vegetables are about twice as likely to develop some types of cancer as those who regularly eat the recommended amounts.

If you want to get the most cancer protection per serving, green vegetables are a great place to start. The cruciferous vegetables, including broccoli, Brussels sprouts, cauliflower, and cabbage are recognized as having special protective effects. These foods contain a naturally occurring cancer-fighting chemical called sulforaphane. People who regularly partake of cruciferous vegetables have a much lower risk of various types of cancer, especially those involving the stomach, colon, and rectum.

The Best Anti-Oxidant Fruits: Grapes

In the fruit department, grapes have recently attained celebrity status.

Grapes are a rich source of an antioxidant called resveratrol. This agent not only helps detoxify cancer-causing free radicals in the body; it also seems to keep tumor cells from invading surrounding tissue.

Eating grapes is beneficial, but drinking grape juice may be even better. Purple grape juice contains double the antioxidant power of many fresh fruits and vegetables. According to the U.S. Department of Agriculture, purple grape juice has more than three times the antioxidants contained in other commonly consumed juices, including grapefruit, orange, tomato, and apple juice.

In a study at Georgetown University, volunteers who drank purple grape juice daily for two weeks experienced a 50 percent increase of antioxidants in their blood levels. They also enjoyed a 30 percent reduction in the production of superoxide, a free radical that contributes to sexual dysfunction by rendering nitric oxide ineffective. Because nitric oxide promotes widening of the blood vessels throughout the body, including the genitalia, it plays a critical role in erection and engorgement during sexual activity.

After just two weeks of consuming the purple grape juice, 70 percent of the volunteers in the Georgetown study showed a dramatic increase in nitric oxide production in their blood. Higher levels of nitric oxide in the body correlate with better sexual function.

Grapefruit

There's no doubt that grapefruit and its juice can be part of a healthy diet: A single serving provides 100 percent of the recommended daily allowance for vitamin C. It's also an excellent source of folate, a B-vitamin that helps prevent heart disease and improves sexual performance.

Grapefruit juice carries the American Heart Association's official stamp of approval. It contains compounds that lower cholesterol levels and reduce the risk for cardiovascular disease and some types of cancer. A Canadian study recently found that grapefruit juice could prevent the growth of breast cancer cells in rodents. Mice receiving grapefruit juice in place of drinking water developed 50 percent fewer breast tumors than water-drinking mice, and those tumors were significantly less likely to spread throughout their bodies.

With all this good news, you may be tempted to drink up. But there's a downside to guzzling grapefruit juice. Several studies have demonstrated that a specific compound in grapefruit, called naringin, has a profound impact on how the body absorbs and degrades certain medications. Drinking just one cup of grapefruit juice can lead to a whopping ninefold increase in the concentration of certain drugs in the bloodstream. Among the drugs found to react to grapefruit juice are many calcium-channel blockers used to treat hypertension and heart disease; some hormones; antihistamines; sedatives; and several of the statin drugs used in the treatment of high cholesterol levels. Even at normal levels, all of these drugs have the potential to interfere with sexual function.

Not only does grapefruit juice increase the concentration of certain drugs in the bloodstream; it also delays their elimination from the body. Both actions can increase the frequency and intensity of the medications' side effects. If you're taking a drug that is likely to interfere with libido or sexual function, these side effects can prove to be devastating for your sex life.

Cranberries

For many women and some men, recurrent urinary tract infections can lead to urinary incontinence and make sexual intercourse uncomfortable or practically unbearable. One doctor-approved home remedy for warding off urinary tract infections is cranberry juice. Cranberries are rich in condensed tannins, chemicals that significantly reduce the number of bacteria responsible for causing the infections. Harvard researchers found that when women consumed cranberry juice daily for six months, they developed 58 percent fewer urinary tract infections than those who didn't.

Cranberries are also being praised for their protective properties against heart disease. Flavonoids in the fruit prevent the oxidation of cholesterol, a process that can damage blood vessels and lead to heart attacks and sexual dysfunction. The oil from the cranberry seed is rich in heart-healthy omega-three fatty acids and vitamin E—compounds known to play important roles in reproductive and sexual health.

Tomatoes

An apple a day may help keep the doctor away, but when it comes to sexual health, the tomato may be the real superstar. Tomatoes have always been part of a healthy diet—they're loaded with B vitamins, vitamin C, and iron. The latest research shows that tomatoes offer more than just good nutrition; they may significantly lower your risk of developing heart disease and prostate cancer.

The yellow jelly surrounding tomato seeds is thought to help reduce the formation of blockages in blood vessels that can lead to heart disease and sexual dysfunction. Researchers in Scotland found that the jelly from just four tomatoes reduced the activity of clot-forming blood cells, called platelets, by up to 72 percent.

Tomatoes may also play an important role in preventing cancer. Scientists believe that the tomato owes its cancer-fighting properties to lycopene, a powerful antioxidant that gives the tomato its vibrant red color.

In women, lycopene-rich diets are associated with a marked reduction in the risk of cervical cancer. In a six-year trial involving nearly forty-eight thousand male health professionals, Harvard researchers found that men who consumed tomato products more than twice a week lowered their risk of developing prostate cancer by as much as 34 percent.

In men diagnosed with prostate cancer, lycopene supplements were found to deter the growth and spread of the disease. Lycopene supplementation also lowered blood levels of prostate specific antigen (PSA), a biological marker commonly used to measure the progression of prostate cancer. These findings offer compelling evidence that lycopene may not only prevent prostate cancer, it may also be useful in the treatment of men who already have the disease.

If you want to add more lycopene to your life, you'll need to add more tomatoes to your diet. Lycopene is abundant in all tomato products, including fresh tomatoes, tomato sauce, paste, ketchup, and salsa. While uncooked tomatoes are loaded with the cancer-fighting ingredient, processed tomato products offer even more. Heat breaks down the cell walls of the tomatoes, making the lycopene easier for your body to absorb.

With all the benefits that fruits and vegetables bring to your health and sexuality, you'll want to pack as many as possible into your diet. Try to eat three to five servings of vegetables and two to four servings of fruit each day. A single serving of vegetables is equal to one cup of those that are raw and leafy; a half-cup of other kinds, whether cooked or raw; and three-fourths of a cup of vegetable juice. A single serving of fruit consists of a medium-size apple, banana, or orange; one-half cup of chopped, cooked, or canned fruit; and three-quarters of a cup of fruit juice.

MEAT, POULTRY, FISH, EGGS, DRY BEANS, AND NUTS

The foods in this group are excellent sources of protein, B-vitamins, iron, and zinc. Dry beans—including soybeans—eggs, and nuts, are similar to meats in providing protein and most vitamins and minerals.

Protein forms the very structure of the human body, accounting for about a fifth of your total weight. Protein is essential to the growth and repair of glands and other tissues, and it is vital to the proper function of every cell, as protein performs some of the most important jobs in the body. Because many enzymes and hormones are actually proteins, they are critical in the regulation of sex hormones and their actions.

Protein is made of smaller compounds called amino acids. There are twenty-two different known amino acids; thirteen of them are considered to be "nonessential," and can be manufactured in the body. The nine remaining "essential" amino acids must be obtained from foods. One such essential amino acid is tryptophan. In the body it is converted to niacin, a B-vitamin important to sexuality, and the neurotransmitter, serotonin, which helps regulate mood and sexual desire.

In general, most animal proteins are considered to be complete, meaning that they contain all of the nine essential amino acids. The incomplete proteins in plant-based foods typically lack one or more of the essential amino acids. By itself, a single vegetable cannot fulfill the body's protein needs, but the combination of plant foods, like beans and rice, provides all the essential amino acids.

Legumes are an excellent source of protein, and when they are combined with grain foods, like rice, wheat, or corn, they meet the body's needs for all nine essential amino acids. They have the added advantage of being high in fiber. Legumes also supply the essential minerals and vitamins necessary for sexual health, including iron, zinc, and the B vitamins. Legumes are an excellent source of complex carbohydrates.

Meat, poultry, and eggs are the highest quality sources of protein available. Animal products are complete proteins that provide the nine essential amino acids. Of course, these foods aren't pure protein; they also contain some fat and cholesterol. Beef is an excellent source of iron and other important minerals and vitamins, but it is a major source of fat for many Americans. Most of us could benefit by selecting leaner cuts, and trimming away visible fat.

Poultry products are sources of high quality protein that are much leaner than beef, especially when their skins are removed before cooking. Poultry meats are rich in vitamin A, a fat-soluble vitamin that is important in the health of the reproductive tract. Like beef, the dark meat of chicken and turkey are good sources of iron, a mineral that is important to healthy red blood cells. Adequate intake of dietary iron helps prevent iron-deficiency anemia, a condition marked by fatigue, low energy levels, and irritability.

As a rule of thumb, two to three ounces of cooked lean meat, poultry, or fish counts as one serving. A three-ounce piece of meat is about the size of a deck of cards. For other foods in this group, one cup of cooked dry beans, two tablespoons of peanut butter, or two eggs count as a third of a serving.

Fish

Fish is an excellent source of protein; it's also low in calories and packed with vitamins and minerals. It is an excellent source of omega-three fatty acids, which are known to help lower blood pressure and cholesterol levels, and ultimately reduce the risk of heart disease and sexual dysfunction. Shellfish are rich in calcium and iodine, a mineral that is known to support proper gland function and hormonal secretion.

As part of a healthy, well-balanced diet, you'll need to include two to three servings of protein-rich foods in your diet every day.

ENVIRONMENTAL
ESTROGENS

While the U.S. meat supply is undoubtedly one of the cleanest and safest in the world, a few consumers and scientists still have a rather large bone to pick with the industry. Over the past several decades, there has been increasing concern about the use of sex steroid hormones in meat-producing animals. Some say that this practice is at least partially to blame for the rise in some types of cancer, infertility, premature onset of puberty in children, and the myriad menstrual and menopausal miseries of many women.

Treatment of beef cattle and other animals with naturally occurring or synthetic hormones is a relatively common practice in the U.S. and Canada. These agents enhance lean muscle growth and improve feed efficiency, making their use a very cost-effective measure for meat manufacturers. In recent years, these practices have been questioned, primarily because no one seems to know for sure if the hormone residues in the meat of treated animals negatively impact human development, reproductive health, or sexuality.

Recent complaints stem from the observation that the U.S. Department of Agriculture's stance that steroid-treated meat is safe for human consumption may be based on weak assumptions and shaky scientific data. Data on hormone levels in beef is based—at least in part—on analyses that are decades old, using technology that is now outdated and possibly less than accurate by today's standards. Some believe that the methods used were not sensitive enough to pick up on the low concentrations of hormone residues in animal tissues. In addition, only limited information on the levels of steroid byproducts and metabolites was considered, when, in fact, these agents may significantly impact humans.

Undoubtedly, the concentration of hormones in the meat that reaches your table is very low, but it is safe to say that even in minute quantities, these steroids may have a negative effect on human health and sexuality. With this in mind, you may want to avoid going overboard in the meat department. Substituting fish, beans, and legumes is an excellent way to supplement the protein and other nutrients offered by a meat-based diet.

Soy

If you're looking for the ultimate health food, soy is a good candidate.

Like most other legumes, soybeans are rich in protein and other essential nutrients. Isoflavones in soy products are powerful antioxidants, capable of disarming dangerous free radicals that trigger many destructive processes in the body, including heart disease, cancer, and sexual dysfunction. Soy-rich diets have been shown to increase laboratory animals' life spans by an average of 13 percent.

Some of the isoflavones in soy, called phytoestrogens, are structurally similar to the female hormone estrogen. These compounds can attach themselves to binding sites in the body normally reserved for human estrogen, shielding susceptible tissues from the hormone's harmful effects. This action comes in pretty handy in the prevention of cancers that are spurred on by estrogen, including cancers of the breast and uterus. Because they behave in a manner that is similar to human estrogen and the estrogen found in hormone replacement therapy, soy phytoestrogens have been shown to significantly reduce many of the symptoms that make menopause so miserable.

Researchers focused their attention on the role of isoflavones in menopause after discovering that Asian women, who typically consume soy-based diets, rarely complain of menopausal symptoms. In one American study, menopausal women placed on soy-rich diets enjoyed a 45 percent reduction in the number of hot flashes they experienced. Soy protein is a good source of calcium, and diets rich in soy have been shown to help ward off osteoporosis in older adults.

Women aren't the only ones who can benefit from the isoflavones in soy products. Asian men eating soy-based diets have a much lower risk of prostate cancer than their American counterparts. Cancer of the prostate gland is triggered by testosterone, and the plant estrogens in soy products seem to help offset some of the destructive actions of this hormone in men. Diets rich in soy protein also help reduce the risk of heart disease and sexual dysfunction by lowering total cholesterol levels by as much as 10 to 20 percent.

The benefits of the little bean can be had with as little as twenty-five grams of soy protein a day, but most experts recommend consuming fifty to seventy grams, the amount contained in about two cups of most soy products. With over twelve thousand soy products now on the market, it isn't as hard to pack soy protein into your diet as you might think. Prepared soy foods, like meat substitutes, baked goods, and nondairy frozen treats, can now be found at most health food stores and many groceries. If you find that you don't enjoy the taste of pure soy foods, you can still add soy milk, soy flour, tofu, or tempeh to your existing recipes.

You can't expect to reap the health benefits of soy if you add it to your diet haphazardly. Isoflavones are easily broken down, and they aren't stored in body tissues. The compounds only remain active in your body for about twenty-four to thirty-six hours.

If you want to keep your body armed with soy power, you'll have to make it part of your daily fare. To make your diet even healthier, you should use soy protein in place of—and not in addition to—the animal proteins in your diet.

Nuts

Nuts are an excellent source of protein and high-quality fat. As plant foods, they're naturally cholesterol free. Nuts are rich in calories, but they're nutrient-dense. Each serving of nuts packs a powerful protein punch, and is loaded with vitamins and minerals. Most are good sources of B vitamins, zinc, and vitamin E.

True to their reputation, nuts are high in fat. In most varieties, 75 percent of calories come from fat. But the fats found in nuts are the friendly types, including monounsaturated and polyunsaturated fats. Unlike the saturated fats in animal products, like meat and dairy foods, the fats found in nuts won't send your cholesterol levels soaring.

Nuts are rich in compounds known as plant sterols, which block cholesterol absorption in the gut, reducing the risk for heart disease and sexual dysfunction. Plant sterols were once prescribed as cholesterol-lowering drugs; today they're used as the active ingredients in cholesterol-lowering margarine and spreads.

Nuts also contain phytochemicals and flavonoids, powerful antioxidants that are known to play a role in the prevention of many chronic diseases, including heart disease, cancer, and sexual dysfunction. Cashews and Brazil nuts are rich in selenium, a mineral that has been shown to protect against many types of cancer. Hazelnuts and almonds are good sources of folate, a B vitamin found to ward off both cancer and heart disease.

Nuts are good sources of arginine, an amino acid that benefits your cardiovascular and sexual health. Arginine is known to play an important role in the relaxation of the blood vessels of the genitalia, facilitating erection and engorgement.

Despite growing evidence that eating nuts can improve your health, many folks shy away from the tasty morsels because of their fat and calorie content. Although an ounce of nuts contains around two hundred calories and twenty grams of fat, adding nuts to your diet doesn't necessarily mean you'll add inches to your waistline.

Because they're high-protein foods, nuts are considered to be part of the meat group. Ounce for ounce, nuts supply roughly the same amount of protein as meat, but when it comes to fiber content, nuts win hands down. Even the toughest piece of shoe-leather meat is virtually devoid of roughage, while nuts are fiber rich. If you're counting calories, it's a good idea to substitute nuts for other protein foods in your diet. Replacing a serving of meat with a serving of nuts is a good place to start.

Eggs

For the past fifty years or so, the American Heart Association has been encouraging people to cut down on their egg consumption. Eggs are cholesterol-rich, and eating them was once believed to dramatically elevate cholesterol levels in humans.

Most of us have tried to comply with the recommended egg-restricting rations, and the egg has become somewhat of a forbidden food. But as it turns out, eggs can be a beneficial part of your healthy diet.

The latest research confirms what many experts have suspected for awhile. If you're reasonably healthy, eating an egg a day won't necessarily drive up your cholesterol level or your risk of heart disease. That's not to say that eggs aren't cholesterol rich. A large egg contains roughly two hundred and thirteen milligrams of cholesterol, about two-thirds of the recommended daily allowance.

If you've never had a problem with your cholesterol, eating an egg or two won't clog your arteries or give you chest pain. If your cholesterol level is higher than you or your doctor would like, you still don't have to swear off eggs altogether. You just have to approach the yolk of the egg with caution, since it contains the entire two hundred and thirteen milligrams of cholesterol, and six grams of fat, to boot. The egg white, on the other hand, is still your benefactor. Two egg whites have just thirty-five calories, and they're totally devoid of fat and cholesterol.

Although the egg has long been vilified, it's actually a rather admirable food, containing a veritable smorgasbord of important nutrients. Each egg has around six grams of protein, providing roughly 12 percent of the recommended daily value for this nutrient. Egg protein is of such high quality that it is often used as the gold standard by which other types of protein are compared.

A single egg contains varying amounts of thirteen vitamins, plus several minerals. The yolk of the egg is one of the few food sources of vitamin D, an ingredient that helps your body absorb calcium and build strong bones.

A large egg packs only about seventy-five calories. If you're still worried about the cholesterol content, you can console yourself with the fact that many of the egg's heart-healthy nutrients, like folate and antioxidants, have important benefits that offset the effects of cholesterol on your heart. Eggs are a good source of zinc, a mineral that is critical to sexual health.

MILK, YOGURT, AND CHEESE

Milk products are excellent sources of protein, calcium, B vitamin, and vitamins A and D. While whole milk and dairy products are naturally high in fat, choosing the low-fat varieties will allow you to get all the calcium you need, without exceeding your fat intake.

You may not drink as much milk as you did as a kid, but getting enough calcium is just as important as it ever was. Men and women need calcium at every stage of life. As a child, you needed calcium to make strong bones and teeth. During adolescence and early adulthood, your body readily absorbs calcium from your diet and packs it into your bones—kind of a calcium savings account for your future. It's important to get enough calcium so that your account will be large enough to support you in your old age.

Around your mid-thirties, your bones reach their maximum size and strength—what experts call "peak bone mass." Your body stops building bones, and simply tries to hold on to its existing bone mass. If you don't get enough calcium as a middle-aged adult, your bone mass—and your calcium account—will begin to dwindle.

Men and women lose bone mass most rapidly in the fifth decade of life, but the process is accelerated in menopausal women when estrogen levels wane. Low-calcium diets speed bone loss even more. If enough bone is lost, osteoporosis develops, and bones become brittle and break easily. Most people realize the importance of calcium when it comes to preventing osteoporosis, but calcium has other health benefits. People who eat calcium-rich diets are less likely to develop high blood pressure than those with calcium-poor diets.

The latest calcium research offers good news for women with premenstrual syndrome (PMS). In a landmark study of over 450 PMS sufferers, supplemental calcium alleviated symptoms like bloating, food cravings, and pain by 50 percent. Dietary calcium has also been shown to play an important role in the prevention of obesity. Researchers at the University of Tennessee recently discovered that high-calcium diets boost metabolism and promote weight loss.

How much calcium do you need? The recommended dosage for premenopausal women and men of all ages is 1000 milligrams a day. Postmenopausal, pregnant, and nursing women need at least 1500 milligrams a day.

Milk and dairy products are the major source of dietary calcium in the U.S. Even low-fat milk and dairy products are calcium-rich, with about 300 milligrams per serving. Shellfish, soy products, and greens are also good sources. The food industry is helping boost calcium intake by fortifying orange juice, bread, and breakfast cereals with extra calcium.

Just meeting your body's need for calcium isn't always enough. You have to avoid foods and beverages that rob your body of calcium. Alcohol and caffeine increase calcium losses in the urine. Since dietary fiber binds calcium and hinders its absorption, so it's not such a good idea to combine high-calcium foods with high-fiber foods. Excessive sodium and protein in the diet waste calcium. Eating a high-salt, high-protein diet can double your calcium needs.

Even if you're eating a calcium-friendly diet, your body may not use the calcium you offer it. Calcium isn't readily absorbed from the adult bowel—your body has to work at it. And it won't even try unless you give it a reason. Weight-bearing exercise, like light weight lifting or walking, is all that most people need to stimulate calcium absorption.

A healthy, well-balanced diet calls for two to three servings of dairy products each day. A serving equals two ounces of processed cheese, one cup of milk or yogurt, one-and-a-half ounces of natural cheese or ice cream, or 1/2 cup of cottage cheese.

FATS, OILS AND SWEETS

Dietary fat has gotten a bad rap lately. It's true that too much fat in your diet contributes to a thousand ills like obesity, heart disease, and some types of cancer, but some fat in your diet is absolutely necessary for your good health.

Fat is found in every cell in your body. It also helps store energy, cushion your internal organs, and keeps your skin soft and supple. Most importantly, fats store and circulate the fat-soluble vitamins A, D, E, and K in your body.

Because fat-free foods don't contain fat-soluble vitamins, a diet that is devoid of fat is nutritionally incomplete and potentially harmful.

Butter, oils, fast foods, junk foods, and the fats in animal products like meat and dairy foods are all good sources of dietary fat. Fatty foods should be eaten with a big dose of moderation, but it isn't necessary to eliminate them completely from your well-balanced diet. Fat should be used sparingly, accounting for no more than twenty to 30 percent of your total daily caloric intake. For most folks, this boils down to a fat intake of about forty-five to sixty-five grams a day. Since fat is hidden in many of the foods that we eat, your best bet is to read the nutrition label to find out exactly how much fat is inside.

Don't be "fat-phobic." Contrary to popular belief, some forms of dietary fat are not only beneficial: They're absolutely essential. High-quality fats help promote good health and ward off a variety of diseases. Of the three main types of dietary fat—polyunsaturated, monounsaturated, and saturated—the polyunsaturated fats are considered to be the most beneficial.

Saturated fats are the bad guys. They usually exist in solid form at room temperature, and they're derived mainly from animal sources, like meats and dairy products. Some plant oils, including palm oil and coconut oil, are also saturated, and they're just as bad for you as animal fats. These fats are often hidden in snack foods, like cookies, cakes, and some types of chocolate. Eating too many saturated fats can elevate your cholesterol levels, leading to clogged arteries and eventually, to heart disease and sexual dysfunction.

Polyunsaturated fats are the good fats. They're liquids at room temperature, and can be found in some plant oils, like sunflower, safflower, soybean, and sesame seed oil. These friendly fats are also found in cold water fish, such as tuna, halibut, herring, sardines, and salmon.

Polyunsaturated oils contain health-promoting substances called essential fatty acids, or EFAs. Because the human body isn't capable of manufacturing these substances, they must be consumed in the diet. Some nutrition experts estimate that roughly 80 percent of American adults consume diets that are deficient in essential fatty acids. Highly processed convenience foods, which make up a large part of the typical American diet, are deliberately stripped of many EFAs to prolong their shelf life.

Diets that are lacking in essential fatty acids can promote or worsen many medical conditions, including diabetes, arthritis, and skin disorders like psoriasis and eczema. Inadequate consumption of these health-promoting substances can aggravate premenstrual syndrome, emotional disorders, and menopausal symptoms.

Recent research suggests that diets rich in EFAs may help strengthen bones and prevent osteoporosis. Essential fatty acids have been shown to increase calcium absorption from the intestines, while reducing excretion of the mineral through the urinary tract.

The essential fatty acids found in fish oils may play an important role in the reduction of breast cancer risk. This protective effect was first observed in Greenland Eskimo women, who thrive on fish-based diets and have extremely low rates of breast cancer.

While diets high in cholesterol and saturated fats are known to contribute to heart disease and sexual dysfunction, diets rich in EFAs have been shown to reduce the risk. The substances lower cholesterol levels, prevent the formation of blood clots in the arteries, and decrease inflammation in blood vessel walls.

As far as your sex life is concerned, EFAs are critical. They are responsible for the function of sex organs, plus the production of sex hormones and adrenal hormones. They also stimulate the production of prostaglandins, hormone-like substances that are so vital to sexual response that they are sometimes injected into the penis to treat erectile dysfunction. Essential fatty acids help maintain healthy circulation and promote the flow of blood to the genitals during sexual arousal and erection.

With the increasing popularity of low-fat and no-fat diets, many Americans have developed an unhealthy fear of fat. Don't let fat phobia cause you to miss out on the friendly fats that are vital to your good health and your sexuality. If you're trying to cut down on your fat consumption, your best bet is to avoid fast food and junk food.

WATER—THE FLUID OF LIFE

Water has no calories, but it is still your body's most important nutrient. Water is vital to life, second only in importance to oxygen. You can survive three weeks or more without food, but probably only about three or four days without water.

As an adult, water makes up about two-thirds of your body, and about 75 percent of your brain. With water as the primary ingredient of your very being, it's easy to see why drinking it is so important. A loss of just 5 percent of your body's water leaves you weak and irritable and impairs your ability to concentrate. A loss of 15 to 20 percent can be fatal.

Your body needs water to stay healthy and fight disease. The mucous membranes that line your nose and throat are your first line of defense against invading viruses and bacteria. When these membranes are moist, they act like flypaper, trapping and destroying germs before they can cause infection. Blood, which is 83 percent water, delivers the cellular soldiers of the immune system throughout the body to help destroy disease-causing organisms.

Water helps lubricate your joints and cushion your organs. It carries food through the digestive system, delivering nutrients and removing waste from cells and tissues. Water washes your eyes and moisturizes your skin.

Water is especially important in terms of your sexuality. As a component of blood, it helps facilitate the delivery of hormones throughout the body, and enhances their effects on target tissues. Adequate water intake is essential for the natural secretions that keep a woman's vaginal lining moist and comfortable. As a primary ingredient of semen, water is important to men's sexual health as well.

Most people lose about ten cups of body water every day. Six cups are lost in urine and feces in the process of waste management. Breathing accounts for an additional loss of two cups each day; water vapor is carried out with each breath you exhale. Approximately two cups of water are lost in the process of cooling your body. Even when you aren't noticeably sweating, water is continuously evaporating from your skin's surface to keep you from overheating. If you exercise, perspiration can lead to the loss of another cup or two.

The average American gets about four cups of water every day without even taking a drink. About three-and-a-half cups are squeezed out of the foods that you eat, and about a half-cup is made as a byproduct of your body's metabolic processes.

Your body relies on fluid intake for the remaining four cups it needs. Most of us offer it everything except what it really wants, and our bodies are faced with the difficult task of extracting water from coffee, tea, and sodas.

If you don't adequately replace your fluids, your body reminds you to do so by signaling to you that you're thirsty. But thirst is an imperfect and rather unreliable signal.

You feel thirsty only after your body is considerably dehydrated, and the salt content of the blood is increased. Salty blood pulls saliva from your mouth, making it feel parched and sending you in search of liquid refreshment. Unfortunately, the thirst signal is easily deactivated. Just wetting your mouth quenches your thirst to a large extent, and most people stop drinking long before they've replaced the fluids that their bodies really need.

Because thirst isn't a reliable indicator of your body's state of hydration, you shouldn't count on it to regulate your fluid intake. Drinking regularly throughout the day is the best way to stay ahead of your fluid requirements.

What your body really wants to drink is plain old water. It doesn't want a beer or a cup of coffee. Alcohol and caffeine act as diuretics, increasing your urine output and partially defeating the purpose of drinking.

Your body doesn't want a soda—the bubbles in carbonated drinks make you feel full and cause you to stop drinking before you've had enough. And because sugary drinks are held in the stomach for digestion, they can't be delivered to the tissues that need them. Water is more easily absorbed and used by the body than any other fluid, and it is the best replacement fluid for your body, bar none.

To date, most studies have shown that bottled water isn't much better—or even different—than plain old tap water. But if shelling out your hard-earned cash for water makes you feel obligated to drink it, then by all means, do it.

Drinking eight glasses of water each day gives you some bonus benefits. You'll be less likely to suffer from constipation, and less susceptible to infections of the upper respiratory tract and bladder. Filling your stomach with water keeps it occupied so that you feel hungry less often and find it easier to lose weight. Drinking water makes your skin look and feel softer and younger.

Water may not be the fountain of youth, but it is definitely the fluid of life. If you haven't had your water today, drink up!

SEXY SPICES

Believe it or not, certain spices are good for your sex life. Here are some to try:

Capsicum

If you like the tingling taste of hot peppers, here's a little good news: Peppers do more than just spice up your food—they can also improve your health and sexual enjoyment. Hot peppers have been used for centuries to add a fiery spark to recipes, and, for just as long, they've been used as aphrodisiacs and medicinal agents. The heat source in hot peppers is capsicum, a remarkably powerful and versatile substance that can be detected in concentrations as miniscule as one part in eleven million.

Consuming peppers can heat up your sex life in more ways than one. Capsicum is known to improve circulation throughout the body. It also helps lower cholesterol levels and decrease the clotting potential of the blood, heading off blockages in the arteries to the heart and genitalia that can lead to heart attacks and sexual dysfunction.

For women prone to develop vaginal yeast infections, here's more good news: Ingredients in hot peppers are toxic to the fungi responsible for causing them.

You probably know from experience that nothing can blast your sinuses clear like a bowl of red-hot chili or a little nuclear salsa. Ingredients in hot peppers are known to stimulate secretions from the mucous membranes. While there are no large-scale studies to prove it, some women report experiencing more copious vaginal secretions after partaking of peppers.

Even if you don't use capsicum for its aphrodisiac or medicinal properties, you and your lover can still share smiles and tears as you tease your taste buds. The firepower that a pepper packs is measured in Scoville units, named in honor of pharmacologist Wilbur Scoville, who pioneered the heat rating system in 1912. The meekest member of the pepper family, the bell pepper, has zero Scoville units, while the average jalapeno packs a whopping 5,500. The hottest pepper in the world, the habenero, weighs in at about 250,000 Scoville units. Think you can handle it? Capsicum is produced by the pepper membranes and then drawn into the seeds. As a rule of thumb, the smaller the pepper, the hotter it tastes, and the greater it's medicinal and aphrodisiac value. Eating the entire pepper, seeds and all, gives you the highest concentration of capsicum, and the most heat. If you enjoy torturing your taste buds, fire away. Hot peppers add more than one kind of spice to your life.

Garlic

Eating garlic probably won't win you the "most popular" award from your friends and colleagues, but when it comes to your sexuality, it might make you a shoo-in for the title of "most likely to succeed." The Chinese have appreciated the medicinal powers of garlic for more than four thousand years, using it to treat a smorgasbord of ailments and afflictions, ranging from indigestion to infection.

One of garlic's greatest virtues may lie in its ability to prevent heart disease. Several studies have demonstrated that regular consumption of the root can lower your total blood cholesterol and triglyceride levels, while boosting levels of heart-healthy high-density lipoprotein (HDL) cholesterol.

Garlic also protects your heart by hindering the clotting ability of your blood. Not only does it promote the formation of clot-busting enzymes, it also diminishes the stickiness of blood cells so that they're less likely to form clots in the first place. Both actions reduce your chances of suffering a heart attack as well as some types of sexual dysfunction. While the anticlotting properties of garlic are beneficial to the sexual and cardiovascular health of most healthy individuals, they can be formidable in folks with bleeding disorders. When it comes to preventing clot formation, hefty doses of garlic can be more potent than aspirin. Before you make garlic a mainstay of your diet, you might want to run it by your doctor.

Regular garlic consumption seems to keep blood vessels more supple and elastic, lowering blood pressure in the process. Some studies have demonstrated that garlic reduces the risk of many types of cancer. In laboratory animals exposed to cancer-causing agents, those who were fed garlic-rich diets consistently developed fewer cancers than the animals who received garlic-free rations.

Several compounds in garlic have powerful antioxidant properties. Antioxidants can disarm dangerous free radicals in the body, agents that are responsible for many of the degenerative changes that inevitably accompany aging. Free radicals are also implicated in triggering cells to mutate and become cancerous. There is evidence to suggest that regular consumption of garlic bolsters the cancer-fighting ability of the immune system by stimulating the production of natural killer cells in healthy individuals. These specialized cells helps prevent the spread of cancer throughout the body. Garlic has long been used as an antifungal and antibacterial agent. Its broad-spectrum antimicrobial properties make it useful in the prevention and treatment of minor yeast and bacterial infections.

You don't have to spend a fortune on packaged or processed pill, oils, and extracts to derive the medicinal benefits of garlic. In fact, fresh cloves of the herb are far more potent that any supplement. And since fresh garlic is usually cheaper, you'll have enough money left over for breath mints.

For most people, the herb is entirely safe and nontoxic in any amount, at least as far as your health is concerned. On the other hand, if the object of your affection finds eau de garlic a real turn off, it can be absolutely lethal to your sex life.

Ginger

Ginger is a very stimulating spice, reputed to stir sexual sensations in the genitalia of men and women. It is known to have anticoagulating properties, capable of increasing the flow of blood throughout the body, including to the sex organs. The roots of the ginger plant can be made into a tea simply by stirring a teaspoon of grated ginger into a cupful of boiling water. You can find pickled ginger in the Asian food section of your grocery, and use it as a condiment to spice up your favorite recipes.

LAST—BUT NOT LEAST—CHOCOLATE!

If you've always known that eating chocolate puts you in the mood for love, now you have scientific evidence to back you up. Chocolate contains phenylethylamine (PEA), a substance found in high concentrations in the brains of people who are happy, in love, or both. PEA is a natural amphetamine, and combines with other chemicals in the brain to produce feelings of excitement, euphoria, and even bliss. Should PEA levels suddenly fall, perhaps as the result of rejection or a breakup, the biochemical consequences are very real. A sudden drop of PEA concentration in the brain can lead to irritability, depression, loss of appetite, and sleeplessness. Many rejected lovers seek solace in chocolate. While chocolate probably won't help bring back the lost love, it can boost PEA levels in the brain, making the symptoms of PEA withdrawal a little more bearable.

Although other foods, including sauerkraut, are richer sources of PEA, chocolate provides an undeniably more palatable—and romantic—package. In animal studies, scientists have discovered that pleasure centers in the brain are activated by chocolate. Although human studies are lacking, most of us don't need additional evidence to convince us that eating chocolate is a pleasurable, sensual experience.

In addition to improving your mood, a piece of chocolate a day may prolong your life. A Harvard study of nearly eight thousand men found that candy consumption was associated with greater longevity. Men who indulged themselves on a regular basis lived almost a full year longer than those who abstained. Chocolate may owe its life-extending properties to antioxidants called polyphenols, which have been shown to lower the risk of developing heart disease. They're also known to protect cells in the body from cancer-causing free radicals. A one-ounce chunk of milk chocolate provides as many antioxidants as most Americans get each day from fruits and vegetables. An ounce of dark chocolate contains twice that amount.

For many people, nothing can take the place of chocolate. That's not surprising, since there is evidence to suggest that the PEA in chocolate can be habit-forming. Chocolate is the most commonly craved food in North America, especially among women—40 percent of women experience cravings on a regular basis, compared to just 15 percent of men. Giving in to those cravings results in a total chocolate consumption of more than twenty-five pounds per person per year.

Since the beginning of time, chocolate has been considered the ultimate edible symbol of love and indulgence. If chocolate puts you in the mood for love, forget about the calories for once, and indulge yourself a little. You can always work them off in the most enjoyable sort of way.

THE NEW SEX HORMONE DIET MEAL PLAN

The Sex Hormone Diet Meal Plan is designed to enhance libido and improve sexual performance in several ways. For starters, it represents a well-balanced, nutritionally complete eating plan, with representatives from each of the five basic food groups. The foods included are rich in the vitamins and minerals that are known to support proper gland function and sex hormone production, as well as amino acids that are necessary for the production of mood-regulating neurotransmitters. These foods are also good sources of energy, and will help revitalize you physically and sexually. Because the diet is rich in essential fatty acids and low in unhealthy types of fat, you can take comfort in knowing that it is as good for your heart and circulatory system as it is for your sexuality.

The aphrodisiac dinners are a little more decadent, so you'll want to save them for special occasions. They're packed with libido-lifting foods, herbs, and spices. You and your lover will enjoy preparing them together, savoring their delectable flavors, and delighting in their sensual aftereffects.

■ DAY 1

Breakfast	Fruit smoothie*
	1 English muffin with raspberry preserves
	Cafe latte with nonfat milk
Lunch	Tomato soup
	Tossed salad with romaine lettuce, cucumbers,
	celery and sunflower seeds with balsamic dressing
	Whole grain roll
	Pear
	Sparkling water with lime
Dinner	Seared tuna steak
	Miso soup
	Vegetable wonton wraps

■ DAY 2

Breakfast	2 Frozen whole-wheat waffles, toasted and topped
	with blueberries and raspberries
	1 Cup of cranberry juice
	1 Cup of milk
Lunch	Greek wrap
	Tabbouleh salad
	Sparkling water with lime
Dinner	Chicken fajitas served with guacamole

---

* Recipes start on page 232.

■ DAY 3

Breakfast	1 Bran muffin with soynut butter
	1 Cup of grape juice
	1 Banana
Lunch	Pita with chicken salad
	1 Orange
	Sparkling water with lime
Dinner	Linguini with clams and garlic sauce
	Steamed asparagus

■ DAY 4

Breakfast	1 Whole wheat bagel with low-fat cream cheese
	1 Cup of orange juice
	1 Cup of grapes
Lunch	Black bean chili
	2 Sesame breadsticks
	1 Banana
Dinner	Grilled salmon with salsa
	Packaged couscous with roasted garlic and parsley

■ DAY 5

Breakfast   Breakfast burrito
1 Apricot
1 Cup of coffee with soy milk

Lunch   Asian chicken salad
1 Cup green tea

Dinner   Beef tenderloin steak
Sweet potatoes
Greens with almond vinaigrette

■ DAY 6

Breakfast   1 Cup oatmeal cooked in low-fat milk and topped
with wheat germ
1 Cup strawberries
1 Cup of grape juice

Lunch   Vegetarian quiche
Low-fat fruit yogurt
Lemonade

Dinner   Ginger lime shrimp kabobs
Grilled eggplant

DAY 7

Breakfast   Apple and cottage cheese toast
1 Cup cranberry juice

Lunch   Tomato, mozzarella, and basil sandwich
1 Small green pepper, sliced
1/2 Cup baby carrots
Sparkling water with lime

Dinner   Vegetable stir fry

SNACKS

Here are some suggestions for healthy snacks to use as part of The New Sex Hormone Diet:

- Frozen yogurt
- Fruit salad: Try a mixture of pineapple, strawberries, grapes, and blueberries.
- Raw vegetables: Cut up a cup of broccoli florets, baby carrots and sliced peppers. Serve with low-fat sour cream dip.
- Toasted whole-wheat bread with cottage cheese and crushed pineapple
- A cup of strawberries in a cup of vanilla-flavored soymilk (instead of cream)
- A healthy snack mix. (See recipe on page 242.)
- Hummus dip with pita chips (See recipe on page 241.)
- Fresh fruit with honey dip (See recipe on page 242.)
- A quarter of a cup of almonds

Aphrodisiac Dinners

SEDUCTION DINNER *1*
• *Raw Oysters* • *Swordfish* • *Garlic Risotto*
• *Sweet Chocolate Truffles*

SEDUCTION DINNER *2*
• *Pork Loin with Spicy Fig Stuffing*
• *Glazed Butternut Squash*
• *Coffee Parfait*

SEDUCTION DINNER *3*
• *Filet Mignon with Truffled Portobello Mushrooms*
• *Fresh Greens with Champagne Vinaigrette*
• *Chocolate Mousse*

SEDUCTION DINNER *4*
• *Boiled Lobster* • *Twice Baked Potato*
• *Fresh Berries and Warm White Chocolate Dressing*

SEDUCTION DINNER *5*
• *Pan-Seared Scallops* • *Penne with Asparagus*
• *Fruit Sorbet*

SEDUCTION DINNER *6*
• *Roasted Garlic Salmon* • *Roasted Vegetables*
• *Peach Melba with Blueberry Sauce*

Aphrodisiac Dinners

SEDUCTION DINNER 7
• *Avocado Soup with Spicy Cucumber*
• *Grilled Sea Bass with*
Kiwi-Mango Salsa • *Spanish Style Cornbread*
• *Lemon-Lime Tequila Sherbet*

SEDUCTION DINNER 8
• *Brandied Beef Medallions*
• *Strawberry Spinach Salad with Almonds*
• *Rum-Ginger Pears*

SEDUCTION DINNER 9
Fettuccine and Clam Sauce • *Garlic Green Beans*
• *Espresso Granita*

SEDUCTION DINNER 10
Gazpacho • *Bruschetta with Fava Beans*

SEDUCTION DINNER 11
• *Provencal Chicken with Rosemary Orzo*
• *Peach and Amaretti Crisp*

SEDUCTION DINNER 12
• *Herbed Roast Leg of Lamb* • *Asparagus and Scallions*
• *Chocolate-Covered Strawberries*

THE RECIPES
(in the order they appear earlier in the book):

FRUIT SMOOTHIE

To make the fruit smoothie, combine the following ingredients in a blender and puree until smooth.

1 cup low-fat vanilla yogurt
1 cup grape juice
½ banana
1 tablespoon honey

TOMATO SOUP

1 12-ounce can tomatoes, diced
1 large onion, finely chopped
3 garlic cloves, minced
½ cup finely chopped basil leaves
1 teaspoon salt
1 teaspoon pepper

In a food processor, combine tomatoes, onion, garlic and basil leaves. Process until smooth. Heat over medium-high heat until warm. Season with salt and pepper.

SEARED TUNA STEAK

Sprinkle tuna steak with salt and pepper on each side. Heat 1 tablespoon olive oil in skillet and then add tuna steak. Sauté over high heat for about 4 minutes. Turn the steaks and brown the other side about 4 minutes longer.

VEGETABLE WONTON WRAPS

⅛ medium head cabbage, finely chopped
⅛ green onion, finely chopped
¼ slice fresh ginger root
¼ water chestnuts, drained and finely chopped
⅛ teaspoon salt
⅛ teaspoon sesame oil
⅛ (14 ounce) package wonton wrappers
3 tablespoons vegetable oil
1 tablespoon and 1¾ teaspoons water

In a medium bowl, mix together the cabbage, green onion, ginger, water chestnuts, salt and sesame oil. Chill in the refrigerator for 6 to 8 hours or overnight. Place a tablespoon of the mixture into each of the wonton wrappers. Fold the wrappers and seal the edges with a moistened fork. In a large, deep skillet, heat 3 tablespoons vegetable oil over medium high heat. Place the pot stickers into the oil seam sides up. Stirring constantly, heat 30 seconds to a minute. Pour water into the skillet. Gently boil 7 to 8 minutes, until oil and water begins to sizzle, then add remaining oil. When the bottoms begin to brown, remove pot stickers from heat.

DIPPING SAUCE

¼ cup soy sauce
¼ cup sesame oil
1 tablespoon of ground ginger

Combine the ingredients in a small serving bowl and stir with a fork.

MISO SOUP

5 cups of water or chicken stock
¼ cup yellow or white miso
¼ cup chopped mushrooms
¼ pound firm tofu, drained and cut into cubes
2 tablespoons sliced green onion

Bring 5 cups of water or chicken stock to a boil and reduce heat to a simmer. Add miso and mushrooms and stir until heated through. Pour into serving bowl and add tofu cubes and green onions.

GREEK WRAP

Spinach tortilla
½ cucumber, diced
1 small onion, sliced
1 small tomato, chopped
1 tablespoon tahini
¼ cup of feta cheese

Lay the tortilla on a cutting board and layer the ingredients. Fold up the bottom quarter of the tortilla and then roll into a cone. Secure with a toothpick.

TABBOULEH SALAD

½ cup medium grain bulgur
1¼ cups water
3 bunches fresh parsley
1½ cups tomatoes, diced
¼ cup green onions chopped

Salt and pepper, to taste

Toss everything together in a bowl. Season with salt and pepper. Chill for about an hour before serving.

CHICKEN FAJITAS

2 large whole boneless, skinless chicken breasts cut in half
1 onion, sliced
2 bell peppers, cut into strips
4 flour tortillas

Season chicken and vegetables with salt, pepper, chili powder, cumin and garlic. Pour 1 tablespoon olive oil in skillet over medium-high heat. Add onions and peppers and cook until they are tender and begin to brown. Remove onions and peppers from heat. Add chicken to skillet and grill on each side for about 6-8 minutes. Wrap tortillas in towel and heat in the microwave for about 1 minute.

Serve with chopped lettuce, low-fat sour cream and guacamole as sides.

GUACAMOLE

1 tomato, chopped
1 clove garlic, crushed
½ cup onion, chopped
2 avocados, pitted and peeled
3 tablespoons lime juice

In a bowl, combine tomato, garlic and onion. Peel and pit the avocado. Scrape the avocado pulp into a separate bowl. Sprinkle with fresh lime juice and mash. Combine mashed avocado with tomato mixture.

PITA WITH CHICKEN SALAD

1 ½ cups minced cooked chicken (use leftover chicken from last night)
½ cup minced celery
¼ cup minced onion
⅛ cup minced pecans
¼ cup mayonnaise
2 teaspoons dill
Salt and pepper, to taste
1 pita pocket

Combine the ingredients. Open pita pocket and fill with chicken salad.

LINGUINI WITH CLAMS AND GARLIC SAUCE

1 tablespoon extra virgin olive oil
2 cloves garlic, chopped
2 tablespoons onion, chopped
18 clams
2 tablespoons white wine
12 ounces linguini, cooked
Fresh basil, chopped

Heat the olive oil in sauté pan. Add garlic and onions and sauté until brown. Add the clams. When shells start to open, add the white wine. Heat the pasta (in salted boiling water), then add to the seafood. Allow pasta to cook in the garlic sauce for a minute, then toss in the basil.

BLACK BEAN CHILI

> 2 teaspoons olive oil
> 1 medium onion, chopped
> 2 garlic cloves, minced
> 1 teaspoon ground cumin
> 1 tablespoon chili powder
> 1 can chicken, beef or vegetable broth
> 1 tablespoon tomato paste
> 2 15-ounce cans of black beans
> Salt and pepper, to taste

Heat olive oil, onion and garlic in saucepan. Cook until onions are soft. Add the ground cumin and chili powder and cook for about 2 minutes. Add the broth, tomato paste and black beans. Reduce to medium heat and let simmer about 30 minutes. Season with salt and pepper.

GRILLED SALMON

> 2 tablespoons Dijon mustard
> 2 tablespoons fresh lemon juice
> 2 tablespoons of choice of fresh herbs
> ½ teaspoon ground black pepper
> 2 (4-ounce) salmon steaks, about 1-inch thick

Combine mustard, lemon juice, herbs and pepper. Brush mixture all over both sides of salmon. Cover with plastic wrap and refrigerate for at least 30 minutes. Place salmon on pre-heated grill or under broiler and cook about 4 minutes per side.

SALSA

> 2 jalapeno peppers
> 1½ cups diced tomatoes
> 2 tablespoons minced onion
> ½ lime, juiced
> Fresh cilantro
> Salt, to taste

Dice the peppers, tomatoes and onion. Chop the cilantro. Combine ingredients in a bowl and season with lime juice. Season with salt, to taste.

Serve salsa over salmon.

ASIAN CHICKEN SALAD

1 broiled or roasted chicken breast, cubed
¼ cup thinly sliced red onions
¼ cup sliced celery
1 lime, juiced
2 tablespoons canola oil
2 tablespoons sesame oil
1 cup romaine lettuce, chopped
¼ cup chopped red pepper
¼ cup chopped yellow pepper
½ cup of raisins
½ cup of cottage cheese

Mix cubed chicken with onions and celery. Combine lime juice, canola oil and sesame oil. Pour over chicken mixture and gently stir. Place on top of romaine lettuce and chopped peppers and sprinkle with raisins. Serve with a side of cottage cheese.

BREAKFAST BURRITO

1 egg
Salt and pepper, to taste
1 teaspoon butter
¼ cup pepper jack cheese
1 flour tortilla

Whisk egg with salt and pepper in small bowl. Heat 1 teaspoon butter in a non-stick skillet over medium-high heat. When butter is melted, add egg and reduce to medium heat. When egg is almost set, add cheese and scramble together by gently turning the egg over and over. Wrap tortilla in a towel and heat in microwave for about 1 minute. Layer egg onto center of tortilla. Fold the top and bottom quarter of the tortilla toward the center and then starting with one side, roll up the tortilla.

BEEF TENDERLOIN STEAK

Enough beef tenderloin for a 3-ounce serving
Pepper, to taste
Tarragon (enough to cover the steaks)
Olive oil

Rub beef with pepper and tarragon. Place skillet over high heat. When hot, using a folded paper towel, carefully wipe surface with olive oil. Place steaks on hot skillet. Cook for about 6 minutes on each side.

SPICY SWEET POTATOES

1 pound sweet potatoes, peeled and cubed
2 tablespoons of honey
3 teaspoons of ginger powder or fresh ginger
2 teaspoons of walnut oil
1 teaspoon of pepper

Toss together sweet potatoes, honey, ginger, walnut oil and pepper. Bake in cast-iron frying pan for 20 minutes in preheated 400-degree oven. Stir potatoes and cook until they are caramelized, about 20 minutes.

ALMOND VINAIGRETTE

Puree the following ingredients for the vinaigrette:

½ cup slivered blanched almonds, toasted until just golden brown
¼ cup olive oil
2 tablespoons freshly squeezed lime juice
1 tablespoon water
½ teaspoon salt
¼ teaspoon freshly ground black pepper

Serve over greens, such as green or red leaf lettuce, romaine or other mixed greens.

VEGETARIAN QUICHE

1 frozen pie shell
1 cup cheddar cheese
1 cup swiss cheese
¼ cup chopped onion
2 jalapeno peppers, chopped
2 tablespoons chopped mushrooms
1 tablespoon chopped parsley
½ cup tofu
4 eggs, beaten
1 teaspoon dry mustard
½ cup sour cream

Layer the cheddar cheese, swiss cheese, onion, jalapeno peppers, mushrooms, parsley and tofu in the pie shell. In a bowl, mix together the beaten eggs, the mustard and the sour cream and pour into shell. Cook at 350 degrees for about 45 minutes.

GINGER LIME SHRIMP KABOBS

12 large shrimp, marinated in lime juice and ginger
1 large onion, sliced into chunks
2 red bell peppers, sliced into chunks
Cherry tomatoes
Salt, pepper and garlic, to taste

Thread ingredients onto skewers, season with salt, pepper and garlic. Place the skewers on the grill and cook for about 3 to 4 minutes on each side. The shrimp should be evenly pink and opaque.

GRILLED EGGPLANT

1 eggplant, sliced
2 small zucchini, sliced
¼ cup peanut oil
2 tablespoons soy sauce

Cut vegetables into half-inch lengthwise slices. Coat with peanut oil and soy sauce. Grill for about 5 to 7 minutes on each side or until all vegetables are tender and well browned.

APPLE AND COTTAGE CHEESE TOAST

1 slice whole wheat bread
¼ cup low-fat cottage cheese
1 fresh apple, sliced
¼ teaspoon cinnamon

Toast bread. Spread cottage cheese on top. Place apple slices on cottage cheese and sprinkle with cinnamon. Place in toaster oven or under broiler until topping bubbles.

TOMATO, MOZZARELLA AND BASIL SANDWICH

2 slices country-style bread
2 slices tomato
2 slices fresh mozzarella
4 whole basil leaves
Pepper to taste
1 tablespoon honey mustard

Layer tomatoes on top of bread slice. Layer mozzarella and basil leaves on top of tomatoes. Sprinkle with pepper. Spread honey mustard on other bread slice and place on top of sandwich.

VEGETABLE STIR FRY

2 tablespoons soy sauce
1 tablespoon oyster sauce
1 tablespoon dry sherry
½ teaspoon white pepper
½ tablespoon sugar
1 teaspoon cornstarch
¼ cup water
1 tablespoon canola oil
1 head fresh broccoli
1 cup snow peas
1 cup sliced mushrooms
1 cup napa cabbage, leaves roughly chopped

In a mixing bowl, combine soy sauce, oyster sauce, dry sherry, white pepper and sugar. To thicken, combine cornstarch with water. Add 1 teaspoon of the cornstarch mixture to the soy mixture until desired thickness is achieved. Set aside.

Peel broccoli stems and cut into small slices. Separate broccoli florets into bite-sized pieces.

In a wok or large skillet, heat canola oil over medium-high heat. Add sliced broccoli stems and cook for 2 minutes. Add broccoli florets, snow peas and mushrooms and cook until tender. Add soy mixture and napa cabbage leaves and cook an additional 1 to 2 minutes.

BROWN RICE

1½ cups brown rice, cooked
¼ bunch of green onions, chopped
1 celery stalk, finely chopped

In mixing bowl, combine cooked rice with green onions and celery. Toss lightly.

HUMMUS DIP WITH PITA CHIPS

1 can chickpeas
¼ cup tahini, well-stirred
2 tablespoons minced garlic
¼ cup fresh lemon juice
Pita bread
Olive oil

Drain can of chickpeas and reserve liquid for later use. In a food processor, puree chick-peas, tahini, minced garlic and fresh lemon juice until hummus is smooth. If needed, add liquid from can of chickpeas to achieve desired smoothness.

Slice pita bread into quarters. Lightly coat with olive oil and broil each side until golden brown.

FRESH FRUIT WITH HONEY-YOGURT DIP

1 cup vanilla yogurt
¼ cup honey
1 teaspoon cinnamon or brown sugar
Fresh fruit, chopped

For dip, combine vanilla yogurt, honey and cinnamon or brown sugar. Serve with chopped fresh fruit.

SNACK MIX

Combine:
1 cup fat-free microwave popcorn, popped
½ cup mini-pretzels
¼ cup cashew nuts
1 tablespoon reduced fat margarine
¼ teaspoon paprika
⅛ teaspoon garlic powder
⅛ teaspoon ground cayenne pepper

OYSTERS

To make the oysters, open 12 fresh oysters, and serve on a bed of crushed ice. Garnish with lemon slices.

SEASONED SWORDFISH

Fresh swordfish filets (about 6 to 8 ounces each, roughly 1½-inch thick)
Olive oil
Salt and pepper, to taste

Heat skillet over high heat. Coat with olive oil. Season swordfish filets with salt and pepper. Add fish to skillet and sauté until lightly golden, about 8 minutes per side.

GARLIC RISOTTO

½ pound orzo pasta
2 tablespoons minced garlic
1 tablespoon olive oil
2 cups chicken broth

Cook orzo and garlic in olive oil until golden. Add chicken broth and cover. Cook over low heat for about 20 minutes.

DARK CHOCOLATE TRUFFLES

10 ounces semisweet chocolate, finely chopped
2 ounces unsweetened chocolate, finely chopped
⅔ cup heavy cream
1 tablespoon of brandy
2 tablespoons unsweetened cocoa, sifted
2 tablespoons confectioner's sugar, sifted

Place the semisweet and unsweetened chocolate into a bowl. Heat the heavy cream over medium heat. Bring to a boil and pour over the chocolate. Whisk until smooth, then whisk in brandy. Refrigerate until firm, but not hard, for one hour.

Line a baking sheet with waxed paper. Using a melon baller, shape the chocolate into ¾ inch balls on the baking sheet. Roll half the balls in cocoa and the other half in confectioner's sugar until completely covered. Store truffles in a sealed plastic container and refrigerate. Remove about one hour before serving.

PORK LOIN WITH SPICY FIG STUFFING

Marinade:
1½ cups freshly squeezed orange juice
¼ cup honey
1½ teaspoons chili powder
½ cup apple cider vinegar
1 tablespoon olive oil
1 pound boneless pork loin

Stuffing:

    2 cups dried figs, chopped
    1 ½ teaspoons chopped roasted garlic
    1 jalapeno pepper, chopped
    4 teaspoons fresh herbs of your choice (such as thyme or parsley)
    ¼ teaspoon salt
    2 tablespoons olive oil with 2 teaspoons lemon zest
    1 teaspoon balsamic vinegar
    ⅓ cup of roasted almonds

Blend together the orange juice, honey, chili powder, vinegar and oil. Pour the marinade over the pork loin in a shallow baking dish, cover and marinate overnight in the refrigerator.

Blend figs, garlic and jalapeno pepper until semi-smooth. Fold in the remaining ingredients.

Remove the pork from the marinade and blot dry. Butterfly the loin lengthwise, leaving ½ inch of meat attached to connect the 2 halves of the loin. Open the pork loin and cover it with plastic wrap. Pound lightly with a butcher's mallet to even thickness, ½ to ¾-inch. Line the stuffing down the center of the loin and fold it closed. Tie the loin carefully at 1-inch intervals with butcher's string.

Preheat oven to 325 degrees. Pour the marinade into a saucepan and reduce it over low heat to a glaze-like consistency. Sear the meat over moderate heat and then roast for 40 to 50 minutes. Brush the pork with the glaze during the last 5 minutes of cooking. Let the meat rest for 5 minutes before removing the string.

GLAZED BUTTERNUT SQUASH

    1 small butternut squash
    ⅛ cup orange juice
    ⅛ cup white cranberry juice
    1 teaspoon cornstarch
    1 teaspoon ground ginger
    ¼ cup water

Cut the squash in half from base and remove seeds. Place halves in baking dish. Cover and bake for 35 minutes in a 350 degree oven. Combine juices, cornstarch, ginger and water, cook and stir over medium heat until slightly thickened. Coat each half of the squash with warm mixture and bake for 10 minutes in 350-degree oven.

COFFEE PARFAIT

> 1 package frozen raspberries, thawed
> ⅛ cup sugar
> 1 tablespoon cornstarch
> 1 cup blueberries
> 2 teaspoons lemon juice
> Coffee ice cream

Drain raspberries. Add enough water to syrup from raspberries to make one cup. Combine sugar and cornstarch. Stir in syrup. Add blueberries. Cook and stir. Bring mixture to a boil. Remove from heat; add raspberries and lemon juice. In wine goblet or any clear glass, layer ice cream and berry sauce.

FILET MIGNON WITH TRUFFLED PORTOBELLO MUSHROOMS

Mushrooms:
> 1 garlic clove, chopped
> 1½ tablespoons butter
> 1½ tablespoons olive oil
> 12 ounces Portobello mushrooms, chopped
> ⅓ cup chicken or vegetable broth
> ⅓ cup dry red wine
> 3 tablespoons whipping cream
> Salt and pepper, to taste

Filet Mignon:
> 1½ teaspoons olive oil
> 2 1-inch-thick filet mignons
> Salt and pepper, to taste
> ½ teaspoon truffle oil

Sauté garlic in butter and olive oil for 30 seconds. Add mushrooms, mix until coated. Cover and cook until mushrooms have released their juices. Add broth, wine and whipping cream and bring to a boil. Cook uncovered until mushrooms are tender and coated with sauce. Season to taste with salt and pepper.

Coat hot skillet with olive oil. Season steaks with salt and pepper. Cook to desired doneness. Place steaks on serving plates. Spoon warm mushroom mixture over steaks and drizzle ¼ teaspoon truffle oil on each.

FRESH GREENS WITH CHAMPAGNE VINAIGRETTE

2 tablespoons Champagne vinegar
1 tablespoon finely chopped onion
⅛ teaspoon mustard powder
1 tablespoon fresh lime juice
½ teaspoon salt
¼ teaspoon black pepper
⅓ cup olive oil

Whisk together vinegar, onion, mustard powder, lime juice, salt and pepper in a small bowl. Add oil in a slow stream, whisking constantly until dressing thickens.

Choose a variety of greens (red leaf lettuce, romaine lettuce and Boston lettuce) and toss with desired amount of dressing.

CHOCOLATE MOUSSE

1 cup chocolate chips
1 egg
1 teaspoon vanilla
1 cup heavy cream
whipped cream

Blend chocolate chips, egg and vanilla in blender. Heat heavy cream until it bubbles at the edges. With blender running, pour in heavy cream. Blend until chips are melted and mixture is smooth. Chill in individual serving dishes and serve with whipped cream.

BOILED LOBSTER

Place 2 lobsters (1½ to 2 pounds each) into a large pot of boiling salted water. Loosely cover pot and cook lobsters over high heat 9 minutes from time they enter water.

Serve with melted butter for dipping.

TWICE BAKED POTATO

2 potatoes
¼ cup sour cream
½ jalapeno, chopped
½ cup grated Monterey Jack cheese
1 finely chopped scallion
salt and pepper to taste

Bake two potatoes. After they've cooled, cut them in half and scoop out the flesh, leaving at least ¼-inch-thick shell. Mash the flesh. Beat until fluffy. Add the sour cream, jalapeno and salt and pepper. Fill shells with mixture. Sprinkle grated Monterey Jack cheese over the potatoes. Bake in 375-degree oven for 10 to 13 minutes. Before serving, sprinkle chopped scallions over each potato.

FRESH BERRIES AND WARM WHITE CHOCOLATE DRESSING

14 ounces white chocolate, cut into chunks
1½ cups heavy whipping cream
3 cups variety of berries (raspberries, strawberries, blackberries)

Melt the chocolate in a stainless steel mixing bowl set over (but not touching) simmering water in a saucepan. Stir until the chocolate is smooth.

Using a wire whisk, add the heavy cream in a steady stream, whisking constantly until it is well incorporated. Continue whisking and adding the cream gradually and the sauce will become completely smooth.

Serve with fresh berries.

PAN-SEARED SCALLOPS

1 tablespoon olive oil
12 sea scallops, patted dry
Salt and pepper, to taste

Heat skillet over high heat, then coat with olive oil. Season scallops with salt and pepper. Add scallops to skillet and sauté until lightly golden, about 4 minutes per side.

PENNE WITH ASPARAGUS

1 pound fresh asparagus
1 teaspoon lemon zest
¼ cup olive oil
½ cup sun-dried tomatoes, chopped
1 pound penne
½ cup parmesan cheese
Salt and pepper, to taste

Cut asparagus into 1-inch pieces, discarding tough ends and setting stems aside. Cook stems in boiling water with salt until tender. Drain stems and transfer to blender. Blanche asparagus tips in same boiling water.

Puree stems with zest, oil and ½ cup of the cooking water. Transfer sauce to a saucepan and add sun-dried tomatoes. Let simmer over low heat.

Cook pasta. Then, add pasta and asparagus tips to sauce and cook over heat, stirring until sauce coats pasta.

Stir in parmesan cheese and salt and pepper, to taste. Cook, stirring, until cheese is melted. Serve immediately.

FRUIT SORBET

Any fruit that you prefer—raspberries and strawberries work particularly well

1 cup orange juice
1 cup champagne
1 lemon, juiced
1 lime, juiced

Place raspberries, strawberries and any other favorite fruits on a baking sheet with wax paper. Store in freezer until all fruit is frozen. In a blender, mix the fruit, orange juice, champagne, and the lemon and lime juices. Freeze in individual dishes until solid.

ROASTED GARLIC SALMON

Garlic puree:
1 head of garlic
¼ cup olive oil
1½ tablespoons unsalted butter
1 teaspoon ground ginger
Salt and pepper, to taste

Salmon:

  2 salmon fillets (6 ounces each)
  2 teaspoons fresh lemon juice
  Salt and pepper, to taste

Slice garlic head in half. Drizzle with olive oil and wrap in foil. Cook in preheated 400-degree oven for about 30 minutes. Scoop or squeeze out softened garlic and puree with oil, butter and ginger. Season with salt and pepper, to taste.

Preheat oven to 450 degrees. Place salmon on baking sheet. Season with salt and pepper. Drizzle each filet with lemon juice, then spread 1 tablespoon garlic puree over each.

Bake salmon uncovered until just cooked through, about 15 minutes.

ROASTED VEGETABLES

  2 small zucchini
  1 eggplant
  2 plum tomatoes
  Salt, pepper and garlic powder, to taste
  Olive oil

Slice zucchini, eggplant and plum tomatoes. Season with salt, pepper and garlic powder. Place on baking sheet, lightly coat with olive oil and bake 30 minutes. Toss once during cooking.

PEACH MELBA WITH BLUEBERRY SAUCE

  1 cup fresh blueberries
  ¼ cup confectioner's sugar
  2 teaspoons fresh lemon juice
  2 peaches, halved and pitted
  Vanilla ice cream or frozen yogurt

Puree fresh blueberries in blender. Stir in confectioner's sugar and fresh lemon juice. Drizzle sauce over serving plate. Arrange halved and pitted peaches on top of sauce. Fill peaches with vanilla ice cream or frozen yogurt.

AVOCADO SOUP WITH SPICY CUCUMBER

1 firm-ripe avocado
1 cucumber, chopped
1 (8-ounce) container plain low-fat yogurt
1 teaspoon fresh lime juice
½ teaspoon chopped fresh jalapeno
1 cup small ice cubes

Peel and pit avocado. Save some for garnish. Blend all ingredients in a blender until very smooth, about 1 minute. Garnish with diced avocado.

GRILLED SEA BASS WITH KIWI-MANGO SALSA

Salsa:

1 kiwi, peeled and chopped
¾ cup peeled and chopped mango
⅔ cup chopped red bell pepper
½ cup diced tomato
⅓ cup chopped cucumber
⅓ cup diced onion
3 tablespoons minced fresh cilantro
2 tablespoons minced seeded jalapeno
2 tablespoons fresh lime juice
Salt, to taste

Sea bass:

6 6-ounce sea bass fillets
Olive oil
Salt and pepper, to taste

Combine kiwi with all ingredients for salsa. Season salsa with salt. Chill to blend flavors.

Prepare barbecue (medium-high heat). Brush fish with oil; season with salt and pepper. Grill about 5 minutes per side. Top with salsa and serve.

SPANISH STYLE CORNBREAD

Add the following ingredients to a standard corn muffin mix:
¾ teaspoon salt
1 teaspoon baking powder
2 tablespoons sugar
1 16-ounce can cream-style corn
1 egg
1 stick butter, melted
½ cup Monterey Jack cheese, cut into chunks
1 teaspoon anise seeds
¼ cup hot water

Pour batter into pan and place the chunks of cheese in the batter, but not fully submerged. Bake about 40 minutes or until golden brown.

LEMON-LIME TEQUILA SHERBET

1 envelope unflavored gelatin
¾ cup sugar
1 cup water
⅓ cup tequila
¼ cup fresh lemon juice
¼ cup fresh lime juice
1 cup vanilla yogurt

Soften gelatin in 2 tablespoons of cold water. Boil sugar and water to make syrup. Let cool. Add gelatin and remaining ingredients. Pour into pan and freeze until slushy. Blend slushy mixture until smooth. Return to freezer. Remove sherbet from freezer 15 minutes before serving.

BRANDIED BEEF MEDALLIONS

¼ cup chopped onion
2 tablespoons olive oil
1 teaspoon molasses
1 cup chicken broth
½ cup beef broth
½ cup brandy
¼ cup whipping cream
2 one-inch-thick beef tenderloin steaks (about 5 ounces each)
Salt and pepper, to taste

Sauté onion in olive oil. Add molasses, stir 1 minute. Add chicken broth, beef broth and brandy. Simmer until sauce is reduced to ½ cup, about 20 minutes. Add cream.

Season steaks with salt and pepper. Coat hot skillet with olive oil. Cook steaks over medium-high heat to desired doneness. Remove steaks. Add sauce to skillet, bring to a boil, scraping up any browned bits. Season to taste with salt and pepper.

Slice steaks and top with sauce.

STRAWBERRY SPINACH SALAD WITH ALMONDS

Dressing:
½ cup sugar
1½ teaspoons chopped onion
¼ teaspoon paprika
¼ teaspoon Worcestershire sauce
½ cup vegetable oil
¼ cup apple cider vinegar

Salad:
Fresh spinach
½ pint fresh strawberries, sliced
⅓ cup sliced almonds, toasted

Mix sugar, onions, paprika, and Worcestershire sauce in a blender. Add oil and vinegar and continue to blend until thoroughly mixed and thickened. Drizzle desired amount of dressing over spinach and strawberries. Add almonds and toss.

RUM-GINGER PEARS

4 cans halved pears
¼ cup brown sugar
1 fresh lemon, juiced
¼ teaspoon of ground ginger
1 tablespoon rum

Arrange pear halves in baking dish, cut side up. Pour pear juice in pan. Combine brown sugar, lemon juice, ground ginger and rum. Spoon mixture into pears and sprinkle with additional ginger. Bake for 15-20 minutes.

FETTUCCINE AND CLAM SAUCE

2 tablespoons olive oil
3 tablespoons minced garlic
1 cup chopped tomato
2 tablespoons chopped parsley
1 teaspoon crushed red pepper flakes
¼ cup dry white wine
2 cans (6 ½ ounce) minced clams. (Drain and reserve liquid in bowl.)
2 cups hot, cooked fettuccine

Heat olive oil in skillet. Add garlic and stir. Add tomato, parsley and pepper. Add wine. Add clam liquid and fettuccine. Toss to coat and cook until liquid evaporates. Stir in clams.

GARLIC GREEN BEANS

2 cups string beans
1 tablespoon minced garlic
1 teaspoon olive oil
1 tablespoon seasoned rice vinegar
1 tablespoon soy sauce

Steam string beans until tender. Chill in ice water, drain and set aside. Sauté minced garlic in olive oil. Add seasoned rice vinegar, soy sauce and green beans. Continue cooking and stirring until hot.

ESPRESSO GRANITA

3 cups strong coffee
1¼ cup sugar
1 cup light cream
1 tablespoon coffee liqueur, such as Kahlua

Heat coffee and sugar. Stir frequently until sugar melts. Remove from heat. Pour in light cream and coffee liqueur. Stir until blended. Let cool. Freeze mixture until hard, about 4 hours. Break into chunks and blend until slushy. Serve in tall glasses.

GAZPACHO

3 cups peeled and chopped ripe tomatoes, or canned plum tomatoes
½ chopped onion
1 yellow bell pepper, chopped
⅔ chopped cucumber
1 cup tomato juice
¼ cup chicken stock
½ teaspoon cumin
1 tablespoon chopped garlic
Pepper, to taste

In a blender, puree tomatoes, onions, half of the chopped yellow bell peppers and cucumbers. Add tomato juice, chicken stock, cumin, chopped garlic and pepper. Whisk until blended. Add the rest of the chopped yellow bell pepper. Refrigerate until well chilled.

BRUSCHETTA WITH FAVA BEANS

1 cup shelled fresh fava beans, cooked and peeled
1 garlic clove, thinly sliced
2 tablespoons black olive paste
8 ounces ricotta cheese
4 thick slices Italian bread, toasted
Extra-virgin olive oil
⅓ cup thinly sliced fresh basil

Combine fava beans, garlic, olive paste and cheese. Top each bread with bean mixture and drizzle lightly with extra virgin olive oil.

VANILLA MINT DIPPING YOGURT

2 cups of low-fat vanilla yogurt
4 teaspoons sugar
⅛ teaspoon vanilla
4 tablespoons fresh mint leaves, thinly sliced
Fruit or sweets of your choice: sliced and peeled kiwis, sliced strawberries,
bananas, almond biscotti, cubed pound cake, etc.

In a bowl whisk together the yogurt, sugar, vanilla and mint. Spoon yogurt mixture into serving bowl. Arrange dippables on a platter alongside serving bowl. Use bamboo skewers or seafood forks as utensils for dipping.

PROVENCAL CHICKEN WITH ROSEMARY ORZO

2 whole boneless chicken breasts with skin, halved
Salt and pepper, to taste
2 tablespoons olive oil
½ cup dry white wine
2 large garlic cloves, minced
White part of 3 leeks, washed and drained well, halved lengthwise, sliced ¼-
inch thick crosswise
2 cups chicken broth
28-ounce can whole tomatoes, drained and chopped
1 teaspoon freshly grated orange zest
1 cup drained kalamata olives, sliced

ROSEMARY ORZO

½ pound orzo
1½ tablespoons extra-virgin olive oil
1½ teaspoons finely chopped fresh rosemary leaves
Salt and pepper, to taste

Pat chicken breasts dry with paper towels and season with salt and pepper. In a large skillet, heat oil over moderately high heat until hot. Brown chicken and transfer to a large plate. Add wine to skillet and boil, mixing in browned bits, until almost evaporated. Add garlic, leeks, broth, tomatoes, zest and chicken. Simmer, covered, turning chicken once, until it is cooked through, about 15 minutes. Transfer chicken to a platter. Add olives to tomato mixture and boil sauce until thickened slightly. Serve over chicken and rosemary orzo.

Bring salted water to a boil in medium saucepan and cook orzo until tender, about 7 to 8 minutes. Drain well and transfer to a large bowl. Toss orzo with oil, rosemary and salt and pepper to taste.

PEACH AND AMARETTI CRISP

Filling:
4 fresh medium-sized peaches, peeled and cut into ¼-inch slices (4 cups)
1 tablespoon granulated sugar
½ tablespoon flour
½ teaspoon vanilla extract

Mix the peach slices with the flour, granulated sugar and vanilla extract. Transfer the mixture to a 2-quart baking dish.

Topping:
½ cup all purpose flour
¼ cup firmly packed light brown sugar
2 tablespoons granulated sugar
½ cup crushed amaretti cookies (about 12)
¾ teaspoon ground cinnamon
¼ cup toasted almonds
6 tablespoons unsalted butter, cut into ½-inch cubes and chilled

In a food processor, pulse together the flour, granulated and brown sugars, amaretti cookies and cinnamon until the cookies are in very small pieces. Add almonds and pulse. Add the butter cubes and continue to pulse until the mixture just begins to stick together. Spread this mixture evenly over the peaches and bake for 30 to 40 minutes, until edges bubble and fruit is tender. Serve warm with vanilla ice cream.

HERBED ROAST LEG OF LAMB

1½ pounds plum tomatoes, sliced thick
7 large mushrooms, quartered
1 red bell pepper, chopped
1 yellow onion, halved
2 fresh rosemary sprigs
2 fresh oregano sprigs
2 fresh thyme sprigs
3 tablespoons olive oil
3-pound leg of lamb, trimmed of excess fat
Salt and pepper, to taste

In a large roasting pan, stir together the tomatoes, mushrooms, bell pepper, yellow onion, rosemary, oregano, thyme and oil. Drizzle lamb with the mixture and season with salt and pepper. Roast the lamb in the middle of a preheated 450-degree oven for 15 minutes, baste with herb mixture, then reduce the temperature to 350 degrees. Cook until lamb registers 145 degrees on a meat thermometer for medium-rare meat. Transfer to a cutting board, cover loosely with foil, and let stand for 15 minutes before serving.

ASPARAGUS AND SCALLIONS

½ pound asparagus, trimmed and lower stalks peeled
10 whole scallions, trimmed and cut to length of asparagus, plus 2 scallion whites, minced
2 tablespoons unsalted butter
Salt and pepper, to taste

Cook asparagus in a saucepan of boiling salted water until crisp-tender, about 5 minutes. Remove asparagus with tongs and immediately plunge into a bowl of ice water. In water remaining in saucepan, cook whole scallions until crisp-tender, about 4 minutes. Remove scallions with tongs and immediately plunge into bowl of ice water. Drain asparagus and scallions on paper towels.

In a large non-stick skillet sauté minced scallion in butter over medium-high heat until softened, about 2 minutes. Stir in asparagus and whole scallions. Salt and pepper to taste and continue to sauté, stirring occasionally, until heated through, about 5 minutes.

CHOCOLATE-COVERED STRAWBERRIES

6 ounces semisweet chocolate, chopped
12 large strawberries

Line small baking sheet with waxed paper. Stir chocolate in top of double boiler set over simmering water until smooth. Remove chocolate from atop water. Dip strawberries halfway into melted chocolate. Gently shake off excess chocolate; place on prepared sheet. Chill until chocolate is set, about 30 minutes and up to 6 hours.

CHAPTER 13

APHRODISIACS:

Pills, Potions, and Promises

THERE ARE HUNDRREDS OF SUPPLEMENTS ON THE MARKET THAT CLAIM to boost libido. A few are worth investigating, and we will explore them here. Others don't live up to the lore. Most of these reuted libido boosters fall into one of four categories: herbs, hormonal compounds, amino acids, or vitamins and minerals. Let's look at herbs first.

HERBAL APHRODISIACS

Before there were synthetic drugs, there were herbs. There's little doubt that many herbs and other natural substances are every bit as effective as "real" medicines, although modern science has a very limited understanding of how most of them work. In spite of the fact that some herbs have been used medicinally for centuries, there is a blatant lack of research concerning their mechanisms of action and even their active ingredients. There's a logical reason for this, if not a good one. Herbs are easily available and surprisingly inexpensive, and there's just no financial incentive to study plant medicines. Synthetic drugs, on the other hand, are required to meet rigid safety standards and efficacy criteria put forth by the U.S. Food and Drug Administration. In meeting these criteria, new prescription drugs are subjected to millions of dollars worth of scientific research. The cost, plus a little extra for the pharmaceutical company coffers, is passed along to the consumer.

If the FDA ever gets around to regulating herbs and supplements, as it has repeatedly threatened to do, more scientific data will become available regarding their actions, benefits, and safety. Unfortunately, if and when this happens, the price of herbs and supplements will climb along with our level of understanding about their active ingredients and modes of action.

In the meantime, our knowledge of how plant medicines work is limited to the odd clinical trial or study, a lot of theories and suppositions, and a tremendous amount of folklore. This leaves us with the challenge of teasing the facts from the fiction, but by applying sound logic to the information that exists, it is possible to draw reasonably accurate conclusions about many of the herbs and supplements that are commonly used.

Although purveyors of herbal aphrodisiacs often allude to the magical or mystical properties of their products, most of us aren't falling for it. Any herb or supplement that claims to be an aphrodisiac is likely to work to improve sexual desire or sexual function in one of three ways: by increasing blood supply to the genitals and facilitating the physical state of sexual arousal; by altering concentrations of neurotransmitters or their effects in the brain; or by influencing hormones or other biochemicals that are known to play a role in sexuality. If the product in question meets one of these criteria, it is likely to have some merit as an aphrodisiac or sexual-performance enhancer, and it may be worth giving a try.

Yohimbine

Yohimbine is derived from the bark of a tree native to the tropical areas of West Africa. For centuries, inhabitants of the region have used the herb to enhance male virility and sexual prowess. Traditionally, West African healers used the inner layers of bark from the yohimbe tree to brew a ceremonial tea. This beverage was used to fuel tribal sex ceremonies that reportedly lasted for up to two weeks. Since its discovery, yohimbine has enjoyed a colorful reputation as a natural aphrodisiac. In an effort to intensify its effects, the herb has been has been eaten, smoked, snorted, and rubbed directly onto the body.

In the early 1980s, the legendary powers of yohimbine sparked the interest of curious doctors and scientists. With the goal of discovering the mechanism behind the magic, a group of researchers set out to study the herb. They eventually succeeded in identifying its active ingredient, a compound now known as yohimbine. Although it was initially speculated that the compound worked by boosting testosterone levels in men, this doesn't seem to be the case. Yohimbine is thought to work in a much more direct manner, simply by increasing the flow of blood to the genital area.

Following a clinical trial conducted by researchers at Queen's University Medical School in Canada, yohimbine gained the respect of the medical community. The results of the study revealed that yohimbine successfully restored erectile function in an impressive 44 percent of men who had developed erectile dysfunction as a result of diabetes and heart disease. Studies like these resulted in the development of several prescription drugs made from yohimbine hydrochloride, now marketed under various brand names, including Yocon, Yohimex, and Aphrodyne. The U.S. Food and Drug Administration has given its seal of approval to these types of drugs for the treatment of erectile dysfunction in men.

Prior to the introduction of Viagra, yohimbine-containing drugs were widely prescribed by physicians. In fact, they were the only FDA-approved medications available for the treatment of the disorder. Even in the era of modern medicine, and in spite of the advent of more sophisticated drugs, the use of yohimbine remains widespread. Natural yohimbine products are available without a prescription in a variety of forms, including capsules, tablets, and tinctures.

If you decide to give the herb a trial run, it's a good idea to discuss it with your doctor ahead of time. Yohimbine can have a stimulating effect, and long-term use of the herb has been reported to increase blood pressure and heart rate. Yohimbine should be used with caution, especially if you have hypertension or any other form of cardiovascular disease. Other side effects of the herb include nausea, headache, anxiety, and flushing. Since concentrations of the active ingredient vary from product to product, you should take the herb as directed by the manufacturer.

Tribulus Terrestris

Tribulus terrestris, also known as "puncture vine" and "goat's head," has been used as an aphrodisiac and medicinal herb for thousands of years. In China, it has primarily been used as a remedy for impotence and other sexual problems, as well as for urinary tract infections.

The herb first hit the Western consciousness in the 1960s, when it was reportedly used by Eastern European Olympic athletes. Because the use of synthetic steroids had been banned, competitors turned to plant medicines and supplements in search of enhanced strength and performance. Tribulus terrestris was credited with increasing muscle mass and strength, primarily by increasing testosterone levels. Several small studies have shown that among men taking the herb, testosterone levels rose by nearly 50 percent.

It is important to note that tribulus terrestris isn't a hormone. It is thought to increase testosterone production in the body by boosting levels of leutinizing hormone (LH), which, in turn, signals the sex glands to manufacture more testosterone.

Several small studies have found that men and women taking tribulus terrestris experience dramatic increases in libido and sexual activity. Use of the plant medicine has been associated with improved sexual performance, more intense orgasms, and greater sexual satisfaction. In women, the herb is thought to alleviate the symptoms of premenstrual syndrome and menopause. In men, it has been shown to increase the quality and quantity of sperm production.

Tribulus terrestris is generally considered to be safe and nontoxic, even when used for extended periods of time. The most common side effect is increased urination. Because the herb has hormone-enhancing effects, it isn't recommended for pregnant women.

Tribulus terrestris can be found in a wide variety of preparations, including tinctures, tablets, teas, and capsules. Since there is no standard of concentration, the potency varies from product to product, and it is advisable to follow label dosage instructions.

Saw Palmetto

Saw palmetto is an herb derived from a dwarf palm tree that grows wild in the southeastern United States. Native American men ate the red-brown berries of the plant to increase sexual vigor and appetite, while women used it to firm their breasts. Saw palmetto yields fatty extracts that seem to be tailor-made by Mother Nature to relieve the symptoms of benign prostatic hypertrophy (BPH). Germany's Commission E, an organization charged with evaluating natural medicines, has given saw palmetto the thumbs-up for the treatment of problems stemming from prostatic enlargement. As a result, German physicians prescribe the herb to more than 90 percent of their patients with the condition. Numerous studies support the effectiveness of saw palmetto in the treatment of BPH. The herb has been shown to double urine flow rates in men with the condition, while halving their number of nighttime bathroom breaks.

Saw palmetto is thought to work its prostatic magic by way of its phytosterols—plant compounds that interfere with the natural hormonal changes that occur in aging men. As men grow older, more of their native testosterone is converted into its roguish hormonal relative, dihydrotestosterone, or DHT for short. Among other things, DHT is responsible for triggering male pattern baldness, the growth of bristly nose and ear hairs, and the enlargement of the prostate gland. Not only does saw palmetto inhibit the conversion of testosterone to DHT, but it also helps block the hormone's ability to act on the prostate gland. The herb's mild anti-inflammatory effects are also thought lessen BPH's symptoms.

The actions of saw palmetto are similar to those of prescription drugs commonly are prescribed to treat BPH's symptoms, but there's at least one critical difference. Saw palmetto causes far fewer side effects, especially the ones that men tend to worry about most: diminished libido and erectile dysfunction. Although saw palmetto effectively alleviates BPH's symptoms, it doesn't actually shrink the prostate gland. For this reason, it's not considered a cure for the condition. Before you take the herb, be sure to talk it over with your doctor. It's possible that your symptoms are caused by something other than an enlarged prostate gland, and you'll want to make sure that BPH is really what you're treating.

Saw palmetto can be taken as a pill or an extract, as well as a tea, and is generally considered to be safe for most people. Because it has steroid-like properties, the plant may interfere with hormone replacement therapies in andropausal men. Saw palmetto is very well-tolerated, and most people don't experience any serious side effects while using the herb.

Ginkgo Biloba

Ginkgo biloba is widely used in traditional Chinese medicine and has recently gained global popularity as a memory booster. More recent research has focused on ginkgo's ability to enhance sexuality, primarily through its ability to increase circulation to the genitals. Although ginkgo biloba is relatively new to the United States, it has been growing in China for more than two hundred million years. The herb, derived from "the tree of good health," has been a major source of traditional remedies for dozens of common ailments for over four thousand years.

Individual ginkgo trees have been known to survive for as long as one thousand years, so it's not surprising that the Chinese believe that the herb derived from it promotes human longevity. Traditional Chinese healers use the extract in the treatment of most age-related disorders. In Germany, where medicinal herbs are available only with a doctor's prescription, ginkgo is approved for use in the treatment of depression, memory loss, and poor circulation.

Scientists still aren't exactly sure how the ginkgo biloba extract works, but they do know that it acts as an anticoagulant substance, hindering the blood's ability to form clots. It also helps dilate blood vessels and improves blood flow to the brain, genitals, and other parts of the body. Both properties are believed to help offset the sexual side effects experienced by many people who take SSRI antidepressants. The herb is thought to have actions similar to those of the prescription drug Viagra.

German scientists recently examined ginkgo's ability to enhance blood flow through the penile arteries. Men with erectile dysfunction were given 60 milligrams of ginkgo biloba extract every day for at least a year. Within eight weeks of starting the supplement, researchers began to note an improvement in blood flow in some of the men. After six months, more than half of the men had regained the ability to achieve an erection.

Ginkgo has long been used as an aphrodisiac; it is reported to have an enhancing effect on desire, excitement, and orgasm. Undoubtedly, the herb's ability to improve blood circulation to the genitals is at least partially responsible for its favorable reputation. There is also evidence to suggest that ginkgo stimulates the production of dopamine, which not only drives the desire for sex, but also heightens the enjoyment that comes from sexual activity. Ginkgo seems to stimulate the activity of the pituitary gland, which ultimately serves to increase testosterone levels.

In a recent trial conducted by scientists at Harvard Medical School, a multi-ingredient ginkgo preparation was found to be particularly effective in the treatment of sexual dysfunction. In addition to ginkgo biloba, the over-the-counter nutritional supplement contained Korean ginseng, Vitamins A, C, and E, and minerals. In the Harvard study, seventy-seven women were asked to take either the supplement or a placebo for a month. At the end of the four-week period, 73 percent of the women taking the supplement reported improvements in overall sexual satisfaction, compared to just 37 percent of those taking the placebo.

In another trial that included thirty men and thirty-three women with SSRI-related sexual dysfunction, volunteer were given sixty to one hundred and twenty milligrams of gingko extract daily. Ninety-one percent of the women and 76 percent of the men taking the herb reported significant improvement in sexual function.

Although traditional Chinese healers brew the nuts of the ginkgo tree into a medicinal tea, most ginkgo products sold in the U.S. are made from the tree's fan-shaped leaves. To date, more than 100 chemicals have been isolated from the ginkgo extract, and it is likely that the mixture, rather than a single agent, is responsible for the herb's wide range of benefits. Ginkgo should be taken on a daily basis to reap all of the sexual benefits that it has to offer. To boost sexual vigor on a more immediate basis, try taking a dose of 180 milligrams about an hour before lovemaking.

Like all herbs, ginkgo is a potentially powerful drug, with equally powerful side effects. While its anticlotting properties are beneficial for most people, they can be hazardous for a few. Taking the herb in combination with other anticoagulant drugs, including aspirin, warfarin, or heparin can be dangerous. At least two ginkgo users have suffered spontaneous bleeding of the brain. Although the herb appears to be safe for most people who aren't taking anticlotting drugs, the consequences of long-term use still aren't known. Other, more common side effects of ginkgo are headaches, feelings of restlessness, skin reactions, stomach upset, and diarrhea. Ginkgo can be found in a variety of forms, including extracts, tinctures, tablets, and teas. Since there is no standard concentration, the potency will vary from product to product, so it is best to follow label directions.

Ginseng

As part of traditional Chinese medicine, ginseng has enjoyed a reputation as a sexual stimulant for more than two thousand years. Ginseng's scientific prefix, "panax," translates to panacea, and, indeed, at one time or another, the herb has been used as a remedy for almost every imaginable type of medical malady. In the hundreds of studies performed to date, there is evidence to suggest that ginseng may have beneficial effects in the treatment of infertility, erectile dysfunction, anxiety, fatigue, hypertension, disorders of the immune system, high cholesterol levels, diabetes, and even cancer. Traditionally, the Chinese used the root of the plant as a general health tonic, believing that it had special powers to replenish energy, forestall aging, and soothe the soul.

In the U.S., ginseng is used for its purported abilities to enhance mood and sexual desire, boost energy levels, and improve sexual and athletic performance. Studies show that it does have a mild stimulant effect, and many people report experiencing improved sexual function after taking the herb. In laboratory studies, male rats taking a daily dose of ginseng were found to experience a twofold increase in testosterone levels. The herb is often given to male breeding animals to improve the quality of their sperm, promote growth of the testes, and foster mating behaviors.

Several active ingredients in ginseng are thought to trigger the production and release of nitric oxide, a substance that is necessary for the attainment of erection in men and clitoral engorgement in women. The herb is known to have estrogen-like effects on the vaginal membranes, making it effective in the relief of the dryness and irritation that often accompany menopause. Many popular herbal preparations include ginseng as an ingredient to help counter the effects of physical and emotional stress. The herb does seem to have stimulatory effects on the immune system and the adrenal glands; both actions can help safeguard the body against stress-related illnesses. Ginseng is also thought to help lower the risk of heart disease and sexual dysfunction by reducing the clotting ability of the blood. Active compounds in the herb interfere with the function of specialized blood cells called platelets, making them less likely to clump together and create blockages.

Most modern herbalists recommend taking the herb for no more than three consecutive weeks, then waiting a week or two before using it again. The Chinese traditionally used the root for short periods of time as well. Taking ginseng for longer periods may lead to overstimulation of the adrenal glands, ultimately rendering them less able to ward off the physical and emotional consequences of stress. To date, there isn't much information regarding the consequences of taking ginseng on a long-term basis, and the herb's potential interactions with prescription medications aren't fully known.

In general, the herb is well-tolerated, as long as it is taken in moderation and according to label directions. Safety concerns center primarily on its ability to interfere with blood clotting. If you're taking other anticoagulant medications, you should ask your doctor about the wisdom of using ginseng products.

Unpleasant side effects primarily arise due to the stimulant properties of the herb. In some individuals, ginseng can cause nervousness, insomnia, and headaches. When combined with other stimulant drugs, blood pressure and heart rate can rise to unpleasant, even dangerous, degrees. Because ginseng has mild estrogen-like effects, the herb may cause breast tenderness and postmenopausal bleeding in some women.

Ginseng comes in a variety of forms, including extracts, tinctures, tablets, teas, and as an edible root. Since ginseng concentrations can vary greatly from product to product, it's important to consult the label for the proper dosage.

Sarsaparilla

Sarsaparilla, sometimes referred to as Chinese root, is native to the Caribbean. Before the advent of artificial flavorings, sarsaparilla was commonly used as an ingredient in a soft drink similar to root beer. It contains hormone-like compounds that resemble natural testosterone, which make it particularly useful as a libido lifter. The root of the plant is also rich in zinc, a mineral that is vital to testosterone production.

Native American women originally brewed the herb into a tea to help expel the placenta after childbirth, and several other cultures have used it to treat "frigidity" in women, and impotence in men. These days, sarsaparilla is used for similar purposes, although some use the herb to help regulate hormones and to boost energy levels.

Sarsaparilla is an ingredient in many natural soft drinks, and it can also be found in the form of an extract or a tincture. The herb is generally considered to be very safe, but taking doses greater than recommended can leave you with an upset stomach. The proper dose varies according to its formulation, so be sure to follow the manufacturer's instructions.

Kava Kava

Kava is a member of the pepper family native to the South Pacific, and has been used by natives of the Polynesian Islands for over three thousand years. Islanders brew the root of the plant into a sacred drink used in rituals. The herb known as the "intoxicating pepper" helps erase sexual inhibitions and create intense feelings of good will. People who take it say that it evokes a sensual feeling of warmth in the genitals. In addition to heightening sexuality, kava kava can induce hallucinations and intoxication.

The active ingredients in the herb are thought to be more than fifteen different compounds known as kava lactones. In the central nervous system, these substances act in a manner similar to prescription mood stabilizers, producing a soothing sense of calm. When taken occasionally and in moderate doses, kava has very few side effects, the most common ones being allergic skin rashes, dizziness, headache, and stomach upset. Although most studies have found that kava does not impair cognitive function, there have been several reports of kava-related citations for driving while intoxicated. If you decide to try the herb, you might want to avoid driving or operating machinery until you see how you tolerate its effects.

Long term use of kava kava has been associated with liver damage and even death, especially in people who regularly consume alcohol. For this reason, the herb should be used only as directed, and only on occasion. When used as an aphrodisiac, kava kava tea should be sipped before lovemaking, but not too far in advance. Its calming effects may make you more desirous of sleep than of sex.

Damiana

Damiana is a small, shrub-like plant native to Mexico, traditionally used as an aphrodisiac and as a treatment for urinary tract infections. Traditionally, Mexican women drank damiana tea prior to lovemaking to increase their sexual receptivity and fertility. The Mayans used the herb to invoke feelings of euphoria. Today, damiana is still used as an aphrodisiac, but it is also found in remedies used to treat menstrual pain and vaginal infections. It is often combined with saw palmetto in herbal preparations designed to promote prostate health and is thought to improve symptoms of erectile dysfunction in men.

Although no clinical studies have examined the effects of the herb, damiana is known to contain compounds that are structurally similar to caffeine. These agents are thought to improve blood flow and sensitivity in the genitals. Like caffeine, the herb has a stimulatory effect that can boost sexual energy. Many users report experiencing a mild state of euphoria for several hours after taking it. Damiana should be taken according to the directions on the package.

Muira Puama

Muira puama, also known as "potency wood," is a small tree that grows in the Brazilian region of the Amazon. Natives of Brazil and Peru have used the root and the bark of the tree as an aphrodisiac for centuries. A recent French study demonstrated the powerful effects of potency wood. Within two weeks of taking the herb, more than 60 percent of the male volunteers suffering from low libido reported improvement, as did more than half of those with erectile dysfunction. Although the mechanism of action remains unclear, muira puama's sexual effects may be attributable to the steroid-like compounds found in the herb.

For its aphrodisiac and performance-boosting benefits, the root of muira puama should be steeped in boiling water and drunk as a tea shortly before lovemaking. When taken as directed, the herb appears to be safe and well-tolerated, with very few side effects.

HORMONAL COMPOUNDS

Believe it or not, the basic building block of all the steroid hormones—including sex hormones—is cholesterol. Although it would seem that by increasing your cholesterol intake, you would be able to increase your body's production of estrogen, testosterone, and other hormones important to libido and sexual function, alas, this isn't the case. Your liver is capable of manufacturing all the cholesterol that your body needs. Any excess is likely to end up blocking your arteries, rather than boosting your steroid levels. As it turns out, the limiting factor in hormone production is usually levels of certain enzymes, rather than cholesterol levels. Judicious consumption of cholesterol is still a good idea, but knowing that it plays at least one beneficial role in your body ought to make you feel a little better about any extra amounts that manage to sneak into your diet every now and then.

Human Growth Hormone

Human growth hormone (GH), also known as somatotropin, is secreted by the pituitary gland in the brain. Secretion of the hormone is normally low until the onset of puberty, when it takes a dramatic upswing, facilitating the changes that occur during the growth spurt of adolescence. By the age of thirty, production begins to slack off a little, and the downhill slide typically persists throughout life. As a strapping young twenty-one-year old, your GH levels were probably in the neighborhood of ten milligrams per deciliter of blood (mg/dL). By the time you reach the grand old age of sixty-one, however, you can expect your levels to have dwindled down to a measly two milligrams per deciliter.

In children and adolescents, release of GH triggers the growth of bones, muscles, skin, and other organs that you've grown accustomed to having. As production of the hormone peters out over the course of adulthood, the same tissues progressively degenerate. As an aging adult, you can expect to end up losing as much as a third of your lean body mass—the nonfat stuff that forms your muscles, bones, and organs. It's also highly likely that your body fat will expand by as much as 50 percent during the same timeframe.

Anti-aging enthusiasts theorize that since aging is caused by the gradual decline in GH, the process can be stopped, and even reversed, by replenishing the substance. Many of them swear that they've found the real fountain of youth in the synthetic version of the wonder hormone. Several studies lend credence to the anti-agers' theory. In a landmark study conducted in 1990, researchers at the Medical College of Wisconsin injected synthetic growth hormone into the bodies of twelve men, ranging in age from sixty-one to eighty-one. By all accounts, the men became stronger, leaner, and more energetic. They felt younger, and some believed that they actually looked younger as well. Many likened the changes in their bodies to turning back the clock ten or even twenty years. This study was the first of thousands to follow; all were intent on discovering the truth about a substance that, at first glance, appears just too good to be true. Interestingly, most subsequent studies have had similar results.

Many adults who yearn to return to their youth are doing just that. They're replenishing their own evaporating supplies of natural growth hormone with a synthetic version of the youth juice. Thanks to recent changes in the U.S. Food and Drug Administration's regulations, the practice is entirely legal, if not universally recommended.

In the past, the use of synthetic growth hormone was approved only in children with a condition known as somatotrophin—or growth-hormone—deficiency syndrome. This condition typically occurs as a result of damage from disease, surgery, injury, or radiation to the pituitary gland, the site of GH production. Growth-hormone deficiency from these causes is rare, affecting only about ten people per million annually in the U.S. On the other hand, a deficiency in GH caused by normal aging eventually affects every single one of us, provided we live long enough. Under the new FDA guidelines, this means that, technically, almost every American over the age of forty now qualifies for replacement therapy.

This is great news for age-defying adults who believe that GH will keep them suspended in a state of eternal youth. In most cases, a six-month course of GH replacement results in a 9 percent increase in lean mass, and a 15 percent decrease in body fat, changes that many of us could definitely use. Users boast of improved exercise tolerance, elevated mood, and less fatigue with exertion. Growth hormone reportedly boosts the immune system, lowers some risk factors for heart attack and stroke, and helps prevent osteoporosis.

It sounds entirely too good to pass up, but before you go galloping back to your glorious youth, there are a few important factors to consider. In most cases, a year's worth of the stuff costs over one thousand dollars, and the price of some treatment regimens can be as much as ten thousand dollars annually. For most folks, that's a pretty big hit, but the drug's price tag may not be its biggest drawback. Not long ago, the National Institutes on Aging (NIA) launched a public service campaign advising consumers to hold off using growth hormone, at least until more is known about it. The organization fears that its use may trigger the development of diabetes, high blood pressure, heart failure, and even cancer. In the meantime, many youth-seeking Americans aren't willing to wait. Thousands are already using GH, and with an ever-increasing number of doctors willing to prescribe it, it's likely that its use will escalate in the future.

DHEA

DHEA, short for dihydroepiandrosterone, is a steroid hormone made from cholesterol in the adrenal glands. These two small organs sit atop the kidneys, and are better known for their production of the hormone, adrenaline. DHEA is the most abundant steroid in the bloodstream, and is present in even higher levels in brain tissue. In the body, DHEA is a precursor to numerous steroid sex hormones, including estrogen and testosterone. Recently, synthetic DHEA has been touted as an anti-aging elixir. It's alleged to remedy almost any ill that ails you, and, more importantly, reverse the aging process.

We all have high levels of DHEA just before we're born, but these levels drop steadily until puberty and then rise sharply, reaching an all-time high when we're in our late twenties. Levels then drop at a rate of about 2 percent per year. If we're lucky enough to reach the grand old age of eighty, our DHEA levels will likely be pitifully low—just 10 to 20 percent what they were in our twenties. DHEA levels fall steadily with age, dropping 90 percent between the ages of twenty to ninety. Since DHEA levels peak during our prime and decline as we age, it's not too farfetched to think that dwindling DHEA levels might have a hand in aging, sickness, and ultimately death.

Although synthetic DHEA replacement therapy has been studied in rodents since 1934, widespread use of the supplement in humans didn't begin until the '90s, when a well-publicized study conducted at the University of California, San Diego, yielded surprising and compelling results. Eighty-four percent of women and 67 percent of men taking supplemental DHEA reported higher energy levels, better sleep, and improved mood. Almost all of the men and women in the study showed an increase in lean body mass and muscle strength, and improved immune function.

This study spawned others, and subsequent claims for DHEA are almost too numerous to count, or to be taken seriously. DHEA has been reported to melt away body fat, and ward off cancer, heart attacks, and Alzheimer's disease. It's said to be useful in the treatment of premenstrual syndrome, diabetes, and osteoporosis. The most alluring claim of all remains its purported ability to reverse the aging process.

A study conducted at the Boston University School of Medicine recently demonstrated that DHEA may help women with some forms of sexual dysfunction. DHEA is a precursor to other biochemicals involved in sexual response, including the hormones androstenedione and testosterone. When a woman's DHEA levels are naturally high, or even adequate, a woman's sex drive is typically strong. But once her levels drop, her desire drops right along with them.

As it turns out, an enzyme present in the adrenal glands, called 17,20-lyase, controls the production of DHEA. In some women, production of this enzyme slows during certain periods of life, including the postpartum period. Falling levels of the enzyme cause levels of DHEA—and a host of other sex hormones—to fall in its wake. This may be the reason that some many women experience a lag in libido after giving birth to their children. While most of us attribute this phenomenon to fatigue and stress, it is possible that low levels of DHEA are at the root of the problem. By taking a supplement, women can override the enzyme deficiency and restore the missing hormone.

A Boston University study evaluated thirty-two women with low androgen levels, all of whom suffered from lack of sexual desire, difficulty becoming aroused, and inability to achieve orgasm. After only six to twelve months of taking fifty milligrams of supplemental DHEA daily, the women reported dramatic increases in sexual desire. They also reported the return of sexual fantasies and the ability to become physically aroused faster and more easily. A study published in the *New England Journal of Medicine* reported that DHEA supplementation improved sexual desire and function in women who had their ovaries surgically removed. Although hundreds of studies have sought to unlock the mysteries of DHEA, no one knows for sure exactly what DHEA does or how it works.

Much of the research regarding DHEA effects has involved rodent subjects, rather than humans. When it comes to DHEA production, rats and mice don't have much in common with humans. Primates, like humans and apes, are the only species that are known to produce large quantities of DHEA, and to demonstrate significant declines in DHEA levels with age. Other animals, including rodents, produce only minute amounts of DHEA. This fundamental difference has left many doctors and scientists wondering if the miraculous effects of DHEA seen in rats and mice will hold true in humans.

On the other hand, researchers have found that DHEA levels are markedly reduced in human beings with almost every major illness or disease, including obesity, diabetes, hypertension, most cancers, and heart disease. Preliminary findings have suggested that supplemental DHEA may help prevent or cure some of these diseases. DHEA has been shown to increase body tissues' sensitivity to the effects of insulin, an action that may help ward off diabetes in humans.

DHEA may have an important role in the prevention of obesity. Men and women taking DHEA show an increase in lean muscle mass. The body's disease-fighting immune system may benefit from DHEA supplementation as well. In one study, women who took fifty milligrams (mg) of DHEA each day had a twofold increase in the destructive activity of their immune cells, and higher levels of potent antitumor and antiviral chemicals.

Until more is known, the potential benefits of DHEA must be weighed against the very real hazards of taking the supplement. Most of the side effects of DHEA are merely annoying, but some researchers claim that DHEA has the potential to be downright dangerous.

DHEA is converted to testosterone in the liver, and most women taking just fifty milligrams of DHEA daily experience a doubling of their normal, physiologic levels of the hormone. For a few women, DHEA causes acne, facial hair, and irregular menstrual periods. In men and women, it can cause male-pattern hair loss and liver damage.

In spite of claims to the contrary, there is no evidence that DHEA prevents cancer. In fact, some experts fear that it may actually stimulate the growth of prostate cancer in men, and increase the risk of breast and ovarian cancer in women. Whether or not DHEA proves to be the real fountain of youth remains to be seen. In the meantime, researchers are working at a fast and furious pace. Until we know more about this super hormone, it should be used with caution, if at all.

Melatonin

Like DHEA, melatonin has been touted as a cure for whatever ails you—from cancer to depression. Advocates of the drug claim that it boosts energy levels and libido, strengthens the immune system, and eliminates insomnia.

Melatonin is a natural hormone produced and secreted by the pineal gland, a tiny, cone-shaped organ that lies at the base of the brain. The pineal gland is known as the "master gland" of the body because it helps regulate all the other glands of the body. It controls the body's biological clock, regulating the rhythms of life. In animals, the gland governs mating, migrating, and hibernating patterns. In humans, its functions are far subtler, but it is the pineal gland that regulates the daily sleep-wake cycle known as the circadian rhythm. The pineal gland communicates with the rest of the body through its hormone messenger, melatonin. Melatonin is manufactured from the neurotransmitter serotonin, which in turn is made from tryptophan, an amino acid derived from protein-based foods.

Melatonin levels peak during childhood and drop during adolescence around the time of puberty. With age, melatonin levels continue to decrease, with the steepest decline occurring around the age of fifty. By the time you're about sixty years old, your pineal gland is producing roughly half the amount of melatonin it did when you were in your twenties. It may be coincidental, but as melatonin levels drop, the body begins to show serious signs of aging. It has been postulated that this drop in melatonin is responsible for aging, and the decline in sexual function that comes with it. It seems logical that by restoring melatonin to more youthful levels, it might be possible to slow some of the deterioration that accompanies the process of growing old.

Whether or not melatonin depletion is responsible for many—or any—of the body's age-related changes is still a subject of great debate. On the other hand, several studies have documented the hormone's ability to regulate the sleep-wake cycle. Melatonin secretion in humans increases as darkness falls and slacks off with exposure to light. Supplemental melatonin has been shown to help reset the internal clock in shift workers and international travelers who suffer from jet lag, and promote sleepiness in people with insomnia.

Melatonin supplements are available in sustained- or immediate-release lozenges, pills, and capsules ranging from half a milligram to 10 milligrams. Because no one knows the normal human level of melatonin, and because it seems to vary from person to person, the therapeutic dose of melatonin is still controversial. Whatever it is, it's probably lower than the dose recommended on the labels of many commercially available products. The dose typically recommended is one to three milligrams before bedtime, but as little as a third of a milligram may be all that's needed if sleepiness is what you're after. Taking more than five milligrams at a time isn't advisable. Melatonin usually causes drowsiness in about thirty minutes, and its effects last for at least an hour. A dose that is too high can lead to daytime sleepiness and a hungover feeling. The short-term side effects of melatonin include vivid dreams, morning grogginess, and headaches. The long-term effects remain unknown.

AMINO ACID SUPPLEMENTS

Amino acids are the basic building blocks of the human body, comprising the muscles, organs, blood cells, and enzymes. Amino acids come in two basic forms: "essential" and "nonessential." Essential amino acids are the ones that human beings aren't able to manufacture single-handedly; they must be obtained from the diet. The human body is capable of producing the nonessential amino acids, although it often requires the presence of other amino acids to use as substrates.

Dietary amino acid supplements are widely popular among bodybuilders and athletes for their muscle-building and strength-generating effects. In theory, the more amino acids delivered to the body via the diet, the faster the production of muscle tissue in response to weight lifting and other forms of exercise. In terms of sexuality, some amino acids seem to help create sex-friendly emotions, while others bring about the requisite biochemical and physical changes in the body. Amino acids are know to elevate mood and energy levels, enhance libido, and promote blood flow throughout the body.

To get the greatest benefit from an amino acid supplement, it should be taken on an empty stomach. This enables it to enter the brain without a great deal of competition from other amino acids. The two amino acids, tyrosine and tryptophan, are known to compete for entry into the brain. The body uses tyrosine to manufacture the excitatory neurotransmitter, dopamine, while it uses tryptophan to make the soothing neurotransmitter, serotonin. If you take a tyrosine supplement after eating a carbohydrate-based food that is rich in tryptophan, you're unlikely to experience any of tyrosine's stimulating or libido-enhancing effects. When it comes to taking amino acid supplements, timing is key.

Arginine

Arginine is an amino acid of the essential variety, so in order to meet your body's needs for the nutrient, you must either consume foods or take supplements that supply it. Until rather recently, arginine was known only for its role in building protein molecules in the human body. The amino acid is a staple in the armamentarium of most bodybuilders, who say that it gives them more energy, stamina, and endurance. They also use it to stimulate the release of the human growth hormone from the pituitary gland, which, in turn, stimulates muscle growth and revs up the metabolic rate, leading to the loss of body fat. The nutrient has also been shown to boost the immune system and speed wound healing.

The hottest area of arginine research centers around its role in human sexuality. In the body, arginine is converted to a simple gas called nitric oxide. In the early 1990s, nitric oxide was pinpointed as the primary mediator of penile erection. The gas is responsible for bringing about the relaxation of blood vessels in the penis, an event that is critical for blood engorgement and erection. Like arginine, some prescription drugs are known to increase nitric oxide concentrations in the penis. Unfortunately, these drugs, which include phentolamine and prostaglandin E1, must be injected into the base of the penis to be effective. Arginine can increase nitric oxide concentrations when taken the easy way—orally.

The supplement seems to work similarly in women, facilitating the clitoral engorgement that comes with sexual arousal. Although large studies are lacking, many women taking the drug report increases in vaginal sensation and secretions. In laboratory studies, female rats given arginine were shown to seek out sexual encounters more frequently and adopt sexually receptive postures more readily. On the other hand, rats deprived of dietary arginine were found to have stunted sexual development.

Arginine may also improve fertility. Livestock breeders routinely give it to their prize bulls, stallions, and roosters to boost their sperm counts. It is also thought to enhance the animals' stamina and endurance, allowing them to withstand the rigors of long breeding seasons.

While arginine is generally safe and well-tolerated, it shouldn't be used by pregnant or nursing women, or by growing children or adolescents. Because the nutrient can influence blood sugar levels, people with diabetes should use it with caution, if at all. You might want to avoid using this amino acid if you have herpes, since it is known to trigger flare-ups and worsen existing outbreaks. If you have the condition and are determined to take arginine, adding a lysine supplement to your diet might be helpful, as lysine is known to inhibit the growth of the herpes virus.

For immediate sex-enhancing effects, a dosage of six to eighteen grams of arginine should be taken about an hour before sexual activity. When used long-term, most manufacturers recommend taking half a gram to two grams, two to three times a day. The recommended dose varies according to body weight and gender, and according to the formulation used. It's always a good idea to follow the manufacturers' directions.

To stimulate the release of growth hormone, the supplement should be taken about an hour before exercise or just before bedtime. To increase the likelihood that the arginine in your supplement will make it to your brain with minimum competition for transport molecules, it's best to avoid eating high-protein foods for a few hours before and after you take the supplement. Good food sources of arginine are poultry and dairy products, Brazil nuts, almonds, peanuts, lentils, kidney beans, soybeans, and sunflower seeds.

Tyrosine

Tyrosine is a nonessential amino acid that the body is capable of manufacturing from phenylalanine. It is known to increase levels of dopamine, a neurotransmitter that plays a critical role in libido, sexual arousal, and orgasm. Low dopamine levels, on the other hand, are associated with depression and diminished sexual desire, as well as with Parkinson's disease. When individuals with Parkinson's disease are given dopamine-boosting drugs, they frequently experience a dramatic increase in sexual interest and sexual behaviors. Tyrosine works by the same mechanism, although when taken at recommended doses, its effects aren't quite as dramatic as those produced by prescription drugs.

Tyrosine is found naturally in meat, fish, dairy, and poultry products as well as in nuts and seeds, wheat, and soy. When taken as a supplement, recommended dosages typically range from 100 to 500 milligrams daily. Most people notice improvements in mood and sexual performance within two to four weeks. Individuals with a history of melanoma shouldn't take the supplement, as it could trigger the growth of any remaining cancer cells. Since it can elevate blood pressure and interfere with glucose metabolism, it should be used with caution in people diagnosed with hypertension or diabetes. To avoid dangerous interactions, tyrosine should not be used simultaneously with antidepressant drugs known as monoamine oxidase (MAO) inhibitors.

VITAMINS

Every vitamin is important for overall health, and ultimately for sexuality. To protect yourself from any deficiencies that might result from a less-than-perfect diet, it's a good idea to take a multivitamin that provides 100 percent of the recommended dietary allowances for each vitamin. If you're interested in boosting your libido and sexual performance, you might want to give extra attention to a few of the standouts.

Vitamin E

Vitamin E has an illustrious reputation as the vitamin of virility. Taking it won't necessarily transform you into sexual superstar, but it is thought to boost human sexuality in several ways. Because it is a critical component in the process of metabolizing food in the diet into energy for the body, it works to enhance sexual energy. Vitamin E is essential for the production of sperm, sex hormones, and gonadotropin, a hormone produced in the pituitary gland that stimulates the production of sex hormones. Studies in laboratory animals show that a deficiency of vitamin E leads to low levels of sex hormones and deterioration of the testes. In test tube studies, vitamin E has been shown to increase the motility of human sperm cells. Other studies have found that the potency and activity of a man's sperm are directly proportional to the amount of vitamin E in his semen. The vitamin may help reduce the risk of cancer of the prostate gland and alleviate symptoms of PMS and menopause.

Vitamin E is one of the most powerful dietary antioxidants known, capable of shielding the body from the deleterious effects of free radicals. As such, it has been shown to play a beneficial role in the prevention of cardiovascular disease. Studies performed at the National Institute on Aging showed that taking vitamin E supplements on a regular basis lowered the risk of heart disease by almost 50 percent. In high doses, vitamin E is reported to slow the progression of Alzheimer's disease, a condition that is caused, at least in part, by the damaging effects of free radicals on brain cells.

Vitamin E appears to help correct the age-related decline in immune system function that puts elderly people at risk for infection. A study published in the *Journal of the American Medical Association* found that taking a daily supplement of 200 International Units (IU) slows the gradual deterioration in immune function that occurs with aging and boosts the body's disease-fighting response to all types of infections. Another study at the NIA showed that subjects who took daily supplements of vitamin E and C reduced their chances of dying from any cause by 40 percent.

The current recommended dietary allowance (RDA) for vitamin E is twelve IU for women and 15 IU for men. Most multivitamin tablets provide 30 IU, but research indicates that daily doses of at least 100 IU units are required to reap the benefits of the vitamin. The risk of toxicity is low, even when much higher doses are taken. Vitamin E is well tolerated by most healthy people, but in those with hypertension, mega doses of the vitamin may elevate blood pressure to a dangerous degree. The richest food sources are vegetable oils and fish oils, eggs, margarine, wheat germ, whole grains, nuts and seeds, and most vegetables, especially green leafy ones.

Choline

Choline is a member of the prestigious family of B vitamins, known best for its essential role in the production of acetylcholine. Acetylcholine is a neurotransmitter that serves sexuality by elevating mood and libido while it facilitates the changes that occur in the body with sexual arousal. Acetylcholine is necessary for the transmission of impulses from the brain to the genital area, which in turn triggers the release of vaginal secretions in women and helps men achieve and maintain erections. If you've ever taken a drug that falls into the anticholinergic class of medications, you probably have experienced first-hand the importance of choline in keeping the mucous membranes of the eyes, mouth, and vagina moist and comfortable.

There is evidence to support the notion that the B vitamin, choline, enhances energy levels and boosts stamina during activity, including sexual activity. It does this primarily by elevating acetylcholine levels. The neuro-transmitter is responsible for sending signals from the nerves to the skeletal muscles throughout the entire body, maintaining proper muscle control and tone.

Several studies have confirmed the importance of choline in facilitating the human sexual response cycle. Too little choline in the diet results in low acetyl-choline levels in the body, which in turn diminishes sexual responsiveness. Acetylcholine is involved in the physical changes that the body undergoes in its journey toward orgasm, as well as the muscular contractions in men and women that make it such a pleasant and memorable event. The neurotransmit-ter also seems to play a role in determining orgasmic intensity and duration.

Laboratory research has shown that the sexual response in females is trig-gered by acetylcholine in the brain. When female rats were given a drug that increased levels of the neurotransmitter in the brain, they exhibited sexually receptive postures. When the same rats were injected with a drug that blocked the neurotransmitter, the friendly posturing ceased.

Although the human body can manufacture small amounts of choline, it doesn't produce an optimal supply, and so this essential nutrient must be obtained from the diet. A choline-rich diet is especially important after the age of forty, when levels of the B vitamin naturally begin to dwindle. Choline is found in lecithin, a fatty acid known to protect cell membranes in the body from damage wrought by free radicals. Lecithin is a major constituent of semen, and it must be replaced after ejaculation.

When used as a libido enhancer or sexual performance booster, choline should be taken about a half-hour before the festivities begin, in doses rang-ing from 100 to 200 milligrams. In some folks, choline is known to impart a fishy body odor, which can definitely be a turn off as far as your sex life is con-cerned. If you're not willing to chance it, you can avoid the fish odor and still reap the benefits of choline by taking a lecithin supplement. Lecithin granules dissolve readily in juice, tea, or soup, and they're not all that bad tasting when they're sprinkled over food. Most manufacturers recommend taking two tablespoons of lecithin daily. Good animal sources of choline include brewer's yeast, egg yolks, liver, fish, meat, and milk. Plant sources of the vitamin include whole grain cereals, beans, peas, nuts, seeds, and green vegetables.

Choline is usually well-tolerated, but it may cause diarrhea in an unfortunate few. It can worsen the symptoms of Parkinson's disease and stomach ulcers, and shouldn't be taken by people with either condition.

Niacin

Niacin is another of the B vitamins, and is vital for healthy skin, proper circulation, and the production of the sex and adrenal hormones. Niacin-containing enzymes in the body play an important role in the metabolism of dietary fats, making it a useful treatment for people with high cholesterol levels.

Folks who take the B vitamin for this reason often experience a dramatic side effect—extreme flushing of the skin. It is this side effect of niacin that makes it valuable as a sex-enhancing tool. Within ten to fifteen minutes of taking it, niacin typically produces warm, tingling sensations that spread throughout the entire body, accompanied by a rosy glow of the skin. This response, called the naicin flush, is remarkably similar to the sexual flush that occurs with lovemaking activities. Both are caused by the release of histamine in the skin, and are entirely harmless. The niacin flush typically lasts for about twenty minutes after taking the vitamin, and can dramatically enhance the pleasure of touch and sexual stimulation, facilitating orgasm.

Niacin is a strong acid, and at higher doses can cause stomach upset in some individuals. People with diabetes, active stomach ulcers, or liver disease should use the vitamin only with their doctor's blessing—and supervision. If you take niacin on a regular basis, your body will quickly develop a tolerance to it, and higher and higher doses will be necessary to trigger the flush. It's best reserved for lovemaking activities, taken in doses of 50 milligrams within fifteen minutes of sexual activity.

MINERALS

Minerals are vital to overall health, not to mention sexual health. They are required for the proper function of every cell in the body, especially those involved in the reproductive process. When it comes to regulating the hormone most intimately tied to libido—and to testosterone—zinc is the most critical.

Zinc

Although zinc serves as a major player in the production of dozens of enzymes involved in thousands of functions, the human body's supply of zinc is relatively small and vulnerable to rapid depletion. The importance of zinc to good health is most apparent when you consider the effects of its absence. In areas of the world where severe zinc deficiencies are common, young boys suffer from delayed sexual maturation and growth retardation. Older men demonstrate low testosterone levels and absence of libido. Men and women of all ages are more susceptible to infections and disease, and often suffer the consequences of delayed wound healing.

While suboptimal levels of zinc can cause sexual dysfunction, a true deficiency can lead to the production of wimpy sperm with poor motility, low sperm counts, and infertility. One of the first signs of deficiency is often a loss of libido. The mineral is necessary for the normal function of the pituitary gland, the master gland of the body that controls all other glands, including those responsible for sexual function. In men, low zinc levels deliver a one-two punch to the sex drive. First, the pituitary gland isn't able to properly signal the testes to produce testosterone— and adequate concentrations of testosterone are necessary to maintain normal zinc levels in body tissues.

Zinc also blocks the actions of aromatase, an enzyme responsible for converting testosterone to estrogen in the human body. With less of the mineral in your system, more testosterone is converted to estrogen. The result is a serious lag in libido and less-than-spectacular sexual performance. Even a mild zinc deficiency can end up having a snowball effect that quickly squashes sexuality in the lustiest of men.

Thanks to the good old American diet, low zinc levels are relatively common in the U.S. Crash dieters, alcoholics, and elderly folks are at greatest risk for zinc deficiency, but even healthy individuals are not immune to the condition. Research has shown that just one month of inadequate zinc intake is enough to reduce testosterone levels by 20 percent. With this in mind, it might not be a bad idea to take a zinc supplement on a daily basis. Several studies have demonstrated that by simply restoring the mineral to normal levels, many effects of its absence are quickly reversed. In one study of men being treated in infertility clinics, the addition of a zinc supplement resulted in significant improvements in testosterone levels and sperm counts in just two months. In healthy men, zinc is concentrated in the semen. Those who engage in sexual activity on a regular basis need to replace the mineral that is lost through the process of ejaculation. Zinc is also concentrated in the prostate and plays an important role in the health of the gland. Several studies suggest that the mineral plays a critical role in regulating the conversion of testosterone to its evil twin, dihydrotestosterone, or DHT. In men, DHT is the hormone implicated in the prostate gland's enlargement, as well as male-pattern baldness. In animal studies, rats placed on zinc-rich diets were found to convert less of their testosterone to DHT.

By now, you're probably convinced that you need to pay more attention to your zinc intake, and you may be right. It's important to make sure that your diet is at least adequate in zinc, but that may be a lot easier said than done. Good sources of zinc include oysters, fish, yogurt, legumes, whole grains, and pumpkin seeds. Absorption from animal foods is far better than from any vegetable source. Since minerals compete with each other for absorption in the body, taking too much zinc can cause you to end up with a deficiency of copper or calcium. It's best to use supplements that offer between fifteen and twenty-five milligrams of zinc, and take one each day to supplement your healthy diet.

CHAPTER 14

ENHANCING ROMANCE

NO MATTER HOW LACKLUSTER YOUR LIBIDO MIGHT BE NOW, there was undoubtedly a time when you were bursting with sexual energy and desire. Back then, expressing your sexuality was as easy as it was important. Remember?

Most people experience the white-hot burn of sexual desire in the early stages of their love relationships, when passion blazes like a wildfire and its ravenous flames consume new lovers. With time, the raging inferno of sexual energy often burns itself out, and the bonfire of romance is reduced to a pile of fading embers.

Think back to the time when you and your partner reveled in the heat of new romance, and when the current of sexual attraction between the two of you crackled and popped—before careers and kids began competing for your time, energy, and affection. Think back to the time before arguments and silences created emotional walls and sexual wastelands. Do you remember the excitement and exhilaration you felt just thinking about your lover? Looking into your beloved's eyes could make your heart stand still and send a million butterflies soaring through your stomach. When you couldn't be alone in private, you whispered passionate promises and sensuous suggestions to each other. When you were apart, you longed to be in each other's arms, and physically ached for each other's touch.

As the intimacy between you began to unfold, you couldn't keep your minds—or your hands—off each other, and you probably made love every time you got the chance. Each sexual encounter was an earthshaking, awe-inspiring revelation that deepened your love and heightened your desire. Even the indescribable physical pleasures of lovemaking couldn't come close to matching the feelings of sheer bliss: the perpetual emotional orgasm that came with being totally intimate and completely connected with your lover.

If you're like most couples, you probably took it for granted that these feelings would last forever. But somewhere along the way, something changed. It might have been so gradual that you didn't even notice it sneaking up. By the time you realized that the passion was gone, you may have found that you and your partner were polarized in your sexual relationship, and the bond that once held you close had become a gaping chasm. Now you may feel trapped and powerless to bridge the gap between you and your lover and incapable of reclaiming the intimacy you once shared.

The first step in reawakening your sexual desire is to explore your feelings about your partner and your relationship. What are the obstacles that are keeping you from expressing and enjoying your sexuality? If you suspect that a medical problem or side effect from a medication is to blame, it's important to see your doctor. If it's a serious emotional issue—like sexual trauma, overwhelming anger, resentment, or distrust—you'll definitely want to consider getting counseling. If your relationship has become a twisting maze of wrong turns and dead ends that leaves you feeling lost and alienat-ed, you may need the perspective of a third party to guide you back and reunite you with your partner.

If you take inventory and find that your feelings about your partner and your relationship are mostly positive, it's a very good sign. If your libido is lame but your love is sound and strong, you'll probably be able to reawaken your sexual desire without professional assistance. It could be that your libido simply got lost in the shuffle of your busy life, and you've been so tired and stressed that you haven't taken the time to look for it. If your sexual desire is suffocating beneath a heap of other responsibilities and commit-ments, it may just need a little resuscitation. As long as your love for your partner is alive and well, the prognosis for the revival of your sexual desire is excellent. With a little time and attention to yourself, your lover, and your relationship, you'll be able to reawaken your desire and rediscover the joys of making love.

MAKE YOUR RELATIONSHIP A PRIORITY

It's completely unrealistic to expect that you'll remain aboard the exhilarating roller coaster ride of newfound love throughout the entire span of your relationship, and this is probably a good thing. If you remained in the lover's limbo that marked the early stages of your relationship, you'd never get anything done. Your house would be a wreck; your career would be stymied; and your friendships would suffer. With sex on your brain all the time, you'd devote all of your time and energy to your relationship, and wouldn't be able to concentrate on anything else.

While it isn't practical to totally abandon life's more mundane responsibilities in your quest to recapture the essence of new love, there is a great deal of merit to the idea of allotting at least some fraction of your time and energy to your sexual relationship. Why did sexual desire come so easily and so naturally in the early stages of your relationship? Was it because you thought about it so often? Most couples admit that, initially, sex was almost always on their minds. If you aren't making love as often as you once did, it may be because you're not thinking about it nearly as often as you used to.

With time, all lasting love relationships grow and mature, and the early feelings of euphoria and excitement give way to emotions that are even better: intimacy and lasting love. On the other hand, even the most mature and intimate relationships can benefit enormously when partners revisit the past and strive to recapture the magic of real romance every once in a while.

The only way to revive your libido and restore your sexual relationship to its rightful position is to make it a priority in your life. Of course, jobs and children demand nearly equal billing, but how about the other things that zap you of your energy and rob you of your time? Is that Saturday morning round of golf or the Tuesday night bridge game more important than your relationship? What good are a manicured lawn and a spotless house if your sex life is in shambles? It's important to maintain your individual interests and to fulfill your obligations, but not at the expense of your most treasured relationship and your sexuality.

If your lack of libido is causing problems in your life, you have to be willing to expend the time and effort necessary to root out the causes and search for the solutions. You have to approach the problem just as you would approach a problem in any other area of your life. Ignoring it will not make it go away: In fact, it will undoubtedly make it worse. You may hope that your diminished desire is just a stage that you're going through, but there's no guarantee that this is the case. It is highly unlikely that you'll wake up one morning and find that your lost libido has mysteriously found its way back to you.

While it may be helpful for you and your partner to discuss the situation when the time and the circumstances are right, if you feel that your loss of libido has more to do with you than your partner, you'll need to take action. You can start by taking a hard look at the priorities in your life. If your sexual relationship is buried beneath a pile of responsibilities including your job, your kids, and your social obligations, it's probably getting only leftover time and attention. While leftover time may be sufficient for some minor details of your life, like cleaning the garage or taking your clothes to the cleaners, it's definitely not nourishing enough to sustain something as important as your sexual relationship with your partner. If your sex life is starving to death on a diet of leftover time, energy, and attention, you'll need to reorganize your priorities and restructure your life. You have to save enough of yourself—both physically and emotionally—to give to your sexual relationship so that it will be properly nourished and nurtured.

Elaine, who operates a successful catering business from her home, admits that she is guilty of starving her sex life. "I'm too busy and too tired to even *think* about having sex. My job is very demanding, and I work long hours—people have parties and weddings in the evenings and on weekends. By the end of the day, I'm ready for sleep, not sex. That's usually when Dave starts coming on to me—when I'm exhausted and sex is the last thing I need. I enjoy making love to Dave, but not when I'm dead tired."

Dave appreciates the fact that Elaine works hard, but he can't help feeling neglected. "She's so busy all the time, baking, talking on the phone, and delivering orders. I feel like her job and her clients always come first. The only time she's ever still is when she's in bed. She just doesn't have any time left to spend with me."

When you structure your life so that time for your relationship is built into your schedule, you'll be less likely to find yourself in situations that involve crisis management. When you're completely exhausted and your partner really wants to make love, it puts you in crisis mode. You have to choose between sleep, which you may desperately want and need, and sex, which you may actually need but don't really want. If you choose sleep, your partner will feel resentful, and you'll feel guilty. If you choose sex, your partner may feel guilty, and you may end up feeling resentful. Neither scenario is exactly a win-win situation, but this self-defeating pattern is incredibly common among couples. It happens because one partner's need for loving, sexual

SUGGESTIONS FOR
SENSUOUS FUN

- Write your lover a love letter or a silly poem.
- Send your lover a formal invitation for a night of romance and lovemaking.
- Plan a picnic under the stars.
- Go for a walk in the moonlight.
- Have sex on your lunch break.
- Take an overnight trip for a little rest, relaxation, and romance.
- Give your lover a luxurious head-to-toe massage.
- Watch a romantic comedy together.
- Make out in the backseat of your car.
- Turn on some romantic music and slow dance with each other.
- Go on an adventure together.
- Meet each other at a restaurant, and pretend that it's your first date.
- Leave a lipstick message on the bathroom mirror.
- Look at old pictures of the two of you, and try to recall and re-experience your feelings for each other.
- Make a videotape about your love for each other for posterity.
- Parade naked through the house.
- Cuddle on the couch.
- Cuddle in bed.
- Sit closer to each other whenever you get the chance.
- Sit on your lover's lap.
- Brush your lover's hair.
- Phone your lover just to say, "I love you."
- Bring your lover a flower.
- Send your lover a greeting card for no reason.
- Play strip poker.
- Make love in every room in your house.
- Read your lover's palm.
- Read love poems to each other.
- Share a meal together.
- Feed each other.
- Rub noses with each other.
- Look deep into your lover's eyes for a full minute.

contact becomes so great that it cannot be ignored, while the other partner feels so tired, stressed, or overwhelmed that the need for love and sexual fulfillment cannot be acknowledged.

To be sure, there will be times in your life when making love gets put on the back burner. For the most part, you can avoid resorting to a style of crisis management by taking a proactive approach. You must find a way to build time into your life for your relationship and your sexuality.

Elaine knew that her long work hours were robbing her of time and energy and hurting her relationship and her sex life. She decided to continue working weekends, but she cut back on the number of evenings that she offered her catering services. "My job is important to me, but not nearly as important as Dave. Now that we have more time to spend together in the evenings, our sex life is back on track."

By making your sexual relationship a priority, you are confirming its importance in your life, and in your partner's. You're conveying your willingness to give of yourself, both emotionally and physically, to nurture the bond between you, and to give it the time and attention that it needs to thrive and grow.

WHAT HAPPENED TO SPONTANEITY?

In the early stages of your relationship, leaving lovemaking to spontaneity was probably a perfectly workable strategy. Romance was always in the air. All it took was a certain look or touch from your lover to ignite your desire and send you scampering off to the bedroom together. But as your relationship matured, and as you both took on new roles and accepted additional responsibilities in life, the spark may have become hidden beneath the myriad layers of your very complex lives. The flickering flames of passion can be easily doused by the distractions of children, career pressures, and hectic schedules. Leaving lovemaking to the whims of spontaneity may no longer be a realistic strategy. Spontaneous lovemaking may not happen often enough to satisfy one or both of you. If this is the case, you'll need to develop a new game plan for your sex life.

Like most couples, Dee and Kyle relied on spontaneity to regulate their sexual activity for the fifteen years that they had been married. Before the birth of their three children, both of them were happy with the arrangement. "Now that I've got three kids and a full-time job, it seems like I never have time for sex. There's always something that must be done, and, usually, making love has to wait. Kyle doesn't seem to understand that—he's constantly badgering me for sex. I know we're not making love as often as we once did, but if I had sex every time he wanted to, I'd never get anything else done."

Kyle saw things from a different perspective. "We hardly ever make love anymore. If I didn't bring it up on a regular basis, we might go for months without having sex." Because Dee usually said no, Kyle felt that he had to ask more often. Kyle resented the fact that he was constantly propositioning his wife for sex, and Dee felt angry and guilty that she was always put in the position of having to turn him down.

When it became obvious to both of them that a spontaneous route to lovemaking just wasn't working, they decided to plan for it in advance. They began to carve out time for lovemaking on the weekends, when their children were usually busy with sports and their friends. Now that they both know that there will be time for romance at least once a week, Kyle doesn't feel like he has to constantly proposition Dee, and Dee feels less pressured and more relaxed.

If you think about it, planning for sexuality makes perfect sense. Most people with busy, productive, and stressful lives leave very few details to chance. You plan your career, your finances, your time, and even your grocery list. But when it comes to one of the most critical aspects of life, too many couples drop the ball. They fail to plan. Why would anyone leave something as important as their sexuality to chance? It's just too important to be cast upon the winds of fate.

With this in mind, you'll need to take a proactive approach to your sexuality, and that involves planning. Planning makes some people nervous, primarily because they aren't accustomed to it. It may seem unnatural, or even a bit too clinical for comfort. Most people who have lost that loving feeling just want it back. They want things to be the way they were. But let's face it: A lot has changed since your relationship was fresh and new. You've changed, your partner has changed, and as a result, your relationship has changed. Your life is complicated. Those young, tender feelings that sprang up in your initial, carefree courtship probably wouldn't survive the rigorous environment of your current relationship. If you're doing nothing but sitting back and hoping for those old feelings to magically resurface, you're in for a long wait. If you're not careful, you may miss your window of opportunity and find that it's too late to recover them.

A STATE OF MIND

As the delightfully insightful Dr. Ruth Westheimer once put it, your greatest sex organ lies between your ears. She's right, of course. Sexual desire starts with a state of mind. This mindset gives rise to sexual thoughts and desires that, in turn, launch dozens of changes in your brain that ultimately trigger the sexual response cycle in your body. While you may have limited conscious control over the physical changes that occur in your body when you make love, you do have enormous control over your state of mind and your thoughts. With a little practice, you can create a sexual state of mind, using your thoughts to fuel your sexual desire. Unfortunately, no one can tell you exactly which thoughts will work best for you. You have to experiment and discover them for yourself. If may take a little trial and error before you learn exactly what works for you, but with patience and persistence, you'll be able to guide your thoughts in a direction that generates sexual desire.

YOUR SEXUAL IDENTITY

Sometimes, sexual desire has less to do with your partner than it does with yourself. It's difficult to muster up the desire for sex when you've lost touch with your sexual identity and when you don't feel sexy. It is important to discover exactly what it is that makes your sexuality tick.

Ron and Linda had been married for fourteen years when they made the mutual discovery that they had lost their sexual identities. Most of their energies were centered around raising their three children. "I thought of myself as nothing more than a mother, and when I looked at Ron, I saw him only as a father to our children."

"We started calling each other 'Mom' and 'Dad' when the kids were young, and it just stuck, even after the children were grown and gone." Ron admits. "It's hard to feel romantic toward someone you call 'Mom.' That was the first thing we changed."

Ron and Linda decided to start paying more attention to their sexuality. For Linda, being sexy had a lot to do with how she dressed. "I threw out all of my granny panties and bought myself some racy lingerie. I don't have the body I used to, but wearing sexy stuff reminds me that there is a sensual side of me. It's not just for Ron; it's for me."

Ron started working out again. "I had really let myself go—I felt like an old man. When I'm in shape, I feel stronger and sexier."

Some people may find that they must create their sexual identities from scratch. Marianne, a thirty-two-year-old mother of two, found herself in this position. "When Adam and I met in college, I was a virgin. We dated for six months before we got married, and I got pregnant on our honeymoon. I really never got a chance to explore my sexuality before the children were born. When the kids were young, I was so busy taking care of them that I didn't have time for much else. My sexuality was a part of me that I had forgotten existed, and I had no idea how important it was to my marriage."

Marianne got a wake-up call when she visited her husband at work. "Adam is a financial officer at a bank, and most of the people he works with are women. I walked into the bank one day and saw him laughing with this young, attractive woman who looked like she had just stepped out of a fashion magazine. It suddenly occurred to me that, compared to her, I looked and acted like a frumpy old housewife. When Adam left for work in the morning, I was still in my pajamas with bad breath and messy hair. By the time he got home from work, I had usually changed into the same old baggy sweat suit. I couldn't remember the last time I had made Adam laugh like that girl at the bank did. I know my husband would never cheat on me, but at that point, I could see how he might be tempted, especially since I had absolutely no interest in having sex."

Marianne decided that she had let herself—and her sexuality—go long enough. "I changed the way I dressed and acted around my husband. I even threw out my favorite sweat suit! I wanted him to find me interesting and attractive. Once I made up my mind to seduce my husband, I couldn't believe how much I enjoyed making love to him. Making Adam crazy is a huge turn-on for me."

Nothing kills libido faster than ignoring your sexual identity. What is it that makes you feel sexy? It's different for everyone. For some, it's an invigorating workout; for others, it's a relaxing massage. It might be wearing your hair a certain way or painting your toenails. It might be reading an erotic novel, watching a romantic movie, or listening to jazz or country music. Whatever it is, do it! Find a way to awaken your sexuality; then nurture it. Give it your time and attention.

Feeling sexy has a lot to do with self-confidence. Remind yourself that you have every right to be confident. If you're in a monogamous relationship, you are the sexiest person in your partner's life. As far as your lover is concerned, you're the hottest thing in town, so treat yourself to a little sexual self-confidence. It's like rocket fuel for your sex drive.

MAKE A DATE

Once your relationship and your sexuality are clearly designated as top priorities in your life, you have to devote a little time and energy to keep yourself from backsliding. It's helpful if you and your partner spend a little time alone each day to mentally reconnect and recommit. A few minutes a day is a good place to start, but it's going to take more than this to keep it going. In mature relationships, sexual desire is dependent on intimacy, and intimacy is not something that can be rushed. There's no shortcut, and you can't achieve it if you're distant, distracted, or uninvolved. Intimacy between two people takes time to develop, and maintaining it depends on spending time together fairly often.

Family time is important, but it doesn't really count as "relationship" time. If you have children, it's just too easy to avoid intimacy by hiding behind your mom and dad roles. It's important to spend time together as a couple. On a regular basis, you should make sure that your kids are well taken care of, and then make a run for it! Relax, have fun, and give your partner your complete attention.

One of the best ways for couples to rekindle the intimacy that they once shared is to establish a weekly "date night." It's hard to give your partner your undivided attention when you're distracted by children or by the endless list of unfinished tasks at home. Sometimes it's best to meet on neutral ground. Taking yourselves away from your home environment helps you see each other as unique individual adults, rather than just as parents or roommates.

Cheryl, a thirty-eight-year-old journalist and mother of three, credits date night with saving her love life. "I work at home, both as a writer and as a domestic goddess. Home is where I spend my time slaving over the computer, the stove, or the washing machine. When I'm there, I feel like I'm at work: I've got a million things to do at any given time. It's hard for me to relax enough to feel romantic, and it's practically impossible for me to feel sexy." She and her husband, Alan, started dating again about a year ago. "Friday nights are special. We put everything else aside: We get out of the house and go do something fun. We make eye contact and conversation and get to know each other better. When I spend time with Alan away from home, it reminds me what an interesting and intelligent guy he is, and I remember why I fell in love with him."

Sometimes it's even better to spend an evening "alone" with friends. Spending time with other couples allows you to showcase your love for each other. It puts you both on your best behavior, and reminds you how you should act for the next week or so. It also lets you view your partner in a different, more flattering light. It lets you see your lover the way other people see him or her, and perhaps the way you once did as well. It shows you the person that you first fell in love with, and brings out the qualities that attracted you to him or her in the first place. It leads you to say, "Ah! That's the person that I fell in love with!" That can be a powerful aphrodisiac.

While Cheryl and Alan like to spend their free time with just each other, Carmen and Marcus found that mingling with other couples on date night worked better for them. "When we went out by ourselves, we always ended up talking about our jobs," Marcus admitted. "We don't do that when we go out with our friends. We have fun with other people, but it's even more fun because we're a couple. When we go out, Carmen always lets me know that she's proud to be with me. She holds my hand and gives me a special little smile that tells me I'm her man. After seventeen years of marriage, I'm still crazy about her." That's the whole purpose of dating—to remind you how crazy you are about each other and to stir up your sexual desire and passion.

Laughter is another powerful aphrodisiac and romance enhancer. When's the last time that you and your mate threw your heads back and laughed together? It is one of the most important things you can do to rekindle your desire for each other. Laughing together creates a special kind of intimacy. Even if you watch a funny movie, or catch a comedy show for a little prepackaged humor, the laughter that results is incredibly powerful. Laughter floods your brain and body with healing endorphins and other neurochemicals that promote feelings of love, facilitate intimacy, and spark sexual desire.

If you and your partner agree that you're not spending enough time with each other and that your sexuality is suffering because of it, dating might help get you back on the right track. Choose a particular night of the week as a standing date night, and keep it as sacred as you can. To make sure that one of you doesn't get stuck with the responsibility of planning the activities every time date night rolls around, try taking turns. See how creative you can make your next outing. It doesn't have to be elaborate or expensive. It can be as simple as taking a moonlit walk, or enjoying a romantic picnic. Even spending the evening at home cuddling on the couch counts, as long as you are alone, free from distractions, and totally focused on each other.

The real purpose of spending time together is to get to know each other better as individuals and to enjoy your relationship as a couple. If it's been a while since you and your partner have spent time together in meaningful ways, you may have an intimacy deficit that needs to be fulfilled before you can move on to higher ground. Be patient. You should strive to reconnect in the pursuit of greater intimacy, and, in doing so, sexual desire will naturally grow and flourish.

If date night leads to lovemaking, that's great. Hopefully, spending a few hours relaxing and reconnecting with your partner will reawaken your desire, and lovemaking will follow as a natural extension of your enhanced intimacy. But if it doesn't happen every time, that's okay, too. The time that you spend together certainly isn't wasted; it is invested. You may not collect on your investment immediately, but eventually it will be returned to you with interest.

THE VACATION MENTALITY

If you find it hard to relax and abandon your endless to-do list long enough to spend time with your partner, you may need to approach your designated time together in the same way that you approach a vacation. Vacations don't just happen; you make them happen. You plan and prepare for them. You take time off from work, wrap things up at the office, and arrange for someone to look after your pets, your house, and your mail. You make travel reservations and secure hotel accommodations. You do all of these things with tremendous anticipation, knowing that you'll be rewarded with fun and relaxation. When you finally lock the door behind you, you start to relax. You make up your mind to leave your worries behind you, because you know they'll still be there when you get back. You surrender yourself to all of the joys and pleasures that come with taking a vacation.

If you can't seem to free your mind and your body from the chains of your day-to-day responsibilities, adopting a vacation mentality toward your sexuality may work for you. Plan and prepare for your time together, savor the anticipation, and then enjoy it with the same abandon that you would enjoy a much-needed and well-deserved vacation.

A CHANGE OF PACE

Making love with your partner should be one of the most pleasurable experiences in your life. If you don't make an effort to keep it sacred and exciting, even this delightful activity can become a chore. You have to work at keeping the romance alive to avoid slipping into a rut. If you and your partner have spent years making love in the same way or the same place, it may be time to expand your sexual horizons. You don't have to do anything that will take you far beyond your comfort zone, but you might be amazed at how much spice a little variety will add to your sexual desire and your enjoyment of lovemaking.

Try varying the place and time of your rendezvous. Plan to meet each other at a motel, or even in your own living room in front of the fireplace. Schedule a meeting by moonlight in your backyard. Take an early lunch and sneak home for a little romance. Turn off the television and take a bubble bath together. If you use a little creativity, your sex life will never become stale. Open up your mind and see where your imagination takes you.

SETTING THE MOOD

Take the time to create a romantic, sensual environment. Send the kids to grandma's house for the evening, turn off the phone and the television, and get ready to relax and enjoy each other. Since each of the five senses is a potential pathway to pleasure, you'll want to titillate as many of them as possible. Light a few scented candles or dim the lights to create a romantic ambience. Excite your lover's sense of sight by wearing something sexy, or perhaps nothing at all. Watch a movie that features steamy love scenes. Visual stimulation triggers the release of brain neurochemicals that heighten your sexual desire and prime you for physical arousal.

Load your stereo system with your favorite CDs. Depending on the mood you wish to create, you can play music that either relaxes or energizes you. Whisper nice or naughty secrets in your lover's ear, or try reading a titillating passage from an erotic novel.

After a relaxing glass of wine, awaken your sense of taste and revitalize your sexual energy by dining on an aphrodisiac meal. Treat your partner's sense of touch to a sensuous massage, and allow your lover to return the favor. Touch releases oxytocin from the brain, and the hormone is known to facilitate bonding and enhance sexual desire. By the time you've stimulated all of your senses, your mind will be fully aroused, and your body will be ready to give and receive all the delightful pleasures that lovemaking has to offer.

RECLAIMING YOUR BIRTHRIGHT

As a human being, you are entitled to sexual fulfillment. The good news is that you can totally revitalize your sexual relationship. You can shake it up and turn it around. You can add the spark that re-ignites the flames of passion between you and your lover, and rekindles the sexual desire that once burned out of control. While you're shoring up the foundation of your sexual relationship, you can add new dimensions and take it to an even higher level. It may take a little time, patience, and love, but the rewards that come with rejuvenating your sexual desire will change your relationship, and even your life. Nothing in the entire human experience is more fulfilling and gratifying than the mutual expression of love and sexuality between two committed people. When you discover what you've been missing, you'll probably wonder why you waited so long to do something about it.

MASSAGE

Take a few minutes to connect with your lover. Speak softly, gaze into each other's eyes, and caress each other lightly. When you're both ready, ask your partner to lie down on his stomach, take a deep breath, and relax. Starting at the temples, gently stroke in circular motions going clockwise, then counterclockwise. Soft touch soothes away tension and enhances relaxation.

Keeping at least one hand on your partner's body at all times, move on to the neck, starting at the base of the head and working down toward the shoulders. Using your thumbs, rub gently downward over the spine. As you move back up, remove your thumbs and allow your fingers to run smoothly up the sides of the neck. Repeat these motions until you feel the muscles begin to relax.

Move on to your partner's shoulders and arms. Start with one arm, and beginning at the shoulder, run your hands down the arm to the elbow and work your way back, rolling the muscles gently between your thumbs and fingers. After massaging the upper arm, use the same motions on the lower arm, stopping at the wrist. Next comes the hand: Massage the back of the hand and the palm, as well as each individual finger. Repeat the entire process on the other arm.

Now turn your attention to the upper back. Start by rubbing gently over the spine, and then sweeping your hands outward toward the arms, and moving downward to the lower back as you go. Continue working from the spine outward. With your thumbs, gently rub the muscles at the top of the buttocks.

One leg at a time, massage the thighs, rubbing the backs and sides in long, sweeping strokes. Move on to the lower leg, focusing first on the calf, and then on the area right above the ankle. Massage the sole of the foot between your hands, including each toe. Using your thumbs, apply pressure as you sweep upward toward the toes. Now that your partner is fully relaxed, it's your turn. Relax and enjoy.

APPENDIX

BARRIERS TO SEXUALITY (BTS)
SELF-TEST

Here is a second copy of the test, designed to help you uncover the problems that may be lowering your libido and preventing you from achieving sexual fulfillment.

Again, the BTS Self-Test has eight phases. Each phase is designed to assess a different aspect of your sexuality. For the questions included in BTS 1 through 35, simply answer "yes" or "no."

Barriers To Sexuality (BTS)
Phase I (Men and Women)

■ BTS 1

Yes	No	Are you a man older than forty-five?
Yes	No	Are you a post-menopausal woman?
Yes	No	Do you have a family history of heart disease?
Yes	No	Do you smoke?
Yes	No	Do you have high cholesterol levels?
Yes	No	Do you have high blood pressure?
Yes	No	Are you sedentary?
Yes	No	Are you overweight?
Yes	No	Do you have uncontrolled diabetes?
Yes	No	Do you experience shortness of breath or chest pain with exertion?

■ BTS 2

Yes	No	Does diabetes run in your family?
Yes	No	Are you overweight, especially around the waist?
Yes	No	Do you have excessive thirst or hunger?
Yes	No	Do you urinate frequently?
Yes	No	Do you have blurred vision?
Yes	No	Do you feel extremely fatigued on a regular basis?
Yes	No	Do you have wounds that are slow to heal?
Yes	No	Do you suffer frequent infections of your skin, urinary tract, or vagina?
Yes	No	Do you experience numbness or tingling of your hands or feet?
Yes	No	Does your mouth frequently feel dry?

■ BTS 3

Yes	No	Do you have diabetes?
Yes	No	Do you eat junk food on a regular basis?
Yes	No	Do you eat red meat more than three times a week?
Yes	No	Do you usually eat whole dairy products instead of the low-fat or reduced-fat varieties?
Yes	No	Do you have high blood pressure?
Yes	No	Are you overweight?
Yes	No	Do you rarely exercise?
Yes	No	Do you have trouble achieving or maintaining an erection (men) or becoming or remaining physically aroused (women)?
Yes	No	Have you had your cholesterol levels checked in the past three years?

■ BTS 4

Yes	No	Are you overweight?
Yes	No	Are you older than thirty-five?
Yes	No	Are you of African descent?
Yes	No	Did your mother or sister suffer a heart attack or stroke before the age of fifty-five?
Yes	No	Did your father or brother suffer a heart attack or stroke before the age of forty-five?

Yes	No	Do you exercise less than thirty minutes a day, three to four times a week?
Yes	No	Do you smoke?
Yes	No	Do you eat more than one teaspoon of salt a day?
Yes	No	Do you drink more than two alcoholic beverages per day?
Yes	No	Do you experience frequent, pulsating headaches?

■ BTS 5

Yes	No	Are you gaining weight for no apparent reason?
Yes	No	Are you unable to lose weight with diet and exercise?
Yes	No	Do you suffer from excessive constipation?
Yes	No	Do you feel cold when others do not?
Yes	No	Do you frequently feel fatigued or sluggish?
Yes	No	Is your hair dry, coarse, breaking, or falling out?
Yes	No	Is your skin dry and scaly?
Yes	No	Do you have puffiness and swelling around your face and eyes?
Yes	No	Do you have difficulty concentrating or remembering things?
Yes	No	Is your sex drive lower than it used to be?

■ BTS 6

Yes	No	Do you feel like your heart is racing or skipping beats?
Yes	No	Do your hands shake?
Yes	No	Do you feel hot, even when others feel cold?
Yes	No	Have you lost weight, even though your appetite is normal or increased?
Yes	No	Do you frequently feel nervous or irritated?
Yes	No	Do you have diarrhea, or loose, frequent bowel movements?
Yes	No	Are you having difficulty getting to sleep, staying asleep, or going back to sleep after awakening in the night?
Yes	No	Do your eyes appear to be larger or more prominent than they used to?
Yes	No	Is your sex drive lower than it once was?
Yes	No	Are you experiencing sexual performance problems?

■ BTS 7

Yes	No	Are you between the ages of twenty-five to forty-five?
Yes	No	Have you had mononucleosis (mono)?
Yes	No	Have you had severe fatigue that has lasted at least six months and does not seem to improve with rest?
Yes	No	Is your fatigue interfering with your daily activities?
Yes	No	Is your throat frequently sore?
Yes	No	Do you have tender lymph nodes in your neck or under your arms?
Yes	No	Do you have joint pain or muscle pain?
Yes	No	Do you have frequent headaches?
Yes	No	Do you awaken from sleep feeling tired?
Yes	No	Do you have fatigue after light exercise or exertion?

■ BTS 8

Yes	No	Has your partner told you that you snore when you sleep?
Yes	No	Have you been told that you stop breathing or gasp for air while you're sleeping?
Yes	No	Are you overweight?
Yes	No	Do you have a thick neck or a double chin?
Yes	No	Do you feel tired and sluggish during the day?
Yes	No	Do you feel as if you could easily take a nap during the day?
Yes	No	Do you have trouble staying awake during the day?
Yes	No	Do you fall asleep unexpectedly during the day?
Yes	No	Are you more irritable than you once were?
Yes	No	Has your doctor told you that you have large tonsils, nasal polyps, or a deviated nasal septum?

■ BTS 9

Yes	No	Do you take a prescription or over the counter medication?
Yes	No	Do you feel that you aren't sure about all of the potential side effects of your medication?
Yes	No	Have you noticed that you feel differently since you began taking your medication?

Yes	No	Have you noticed a decrease in sexual desire since you began taking your medication?
Yes	No	Have you noticed a reduction in sexual performance since you began taking your medication?
Yes	No	Do you find that sex is less enjoyable since you began taking your medication?
Yes	No	Do you drink grapefruit juice one or more times per week?

■ BTS 10 (Women)

Yes	No	Are you older than thirty-five?
Yes	No	Do you suffer from frequent urinary tract infections?
Yes	No	Do you have diabetes?
Yes	No	Are you menopausal?
Yes	No	Have you had more than two children?
Yes	No	Do you drink more than three caffeine-containing beverages a day?
Yes	No	Do you experience loss of urine when coughing, sneezing, or laughing?
Yes	No	Do you feel the need to urinate frequently?
Yes	No	Do you experience a sudden, urgent need to urinate?
Yes	No	Have you had abdominal or pelvic surgery?

■ BTS 11 (Men)

Yes	No	Are you older than fifty?
Yes	No	Do you have trouble starting urination?
Yes	No	Do you have a weak flow of urine?
Yes	No	Do you experience dribbling after urination?
Yes	No	Do you feel that your bladder is not completely empty after urinating?
Yes	No	Do you have the urge to go again soon after urinating?
Yes	No	Do you have pain during urination?
Yes	No	Do you wake at night to urinate?
Yes	No	Do you have frequent urination?
Yes	No	Do you experience sudden, uncontrollable urges to urinate?

Barriers to Sexuality Phase II (Men and Women)

■ BTS 12

Yes	No	Do you feel sad or down most of the day, nearly every day?
Yes	No	Do you have less interest in the activities that you normally enjoy?
Yes	No	Have you lost or gained weight, or noticed a change in appetite?
Yes	No	Are you sleeping too little or too much?
Yes	No	Do you often feel hopeless or worthless?
Yes	No	Do you think about dying or killing yourself?
Yes	No	Do you cry easily?
Yes	No	Do you have trouble remembering things?
Yes	No	Do you have a family history of depression?
Yes	No	Do you have less interest in having sex than you once did?

■ BTS 13

Yes	No	Do you frequently feel sad, angry, or irritated?
Yes	No	Do you suffer frequent upper respiratory infections?
Yes	No	Do you have trouble falling asleep or staying asleep?
Yes	No	Have you had a recent change in appetite?
Yes	No	Do you have less interest in sex than you once did?
Yes	No	Do you feel that your life is getting out of control?
Yes	No	Are you having trouble concentrating or remembering?

■ BTS 14

Yes	No	When you look at yourself in the mirror, are you dissatisfied with your reflection?
Yes	No	Do you find some aspect of your appearance unacceptable?
Yes	No	Do you wear clothes that hide some part of your body?
Yes	No	Do you sometimes avoid certain social events because of your appearance?
Yes	No	Do you feel that you spend too much time worrying about your weight or appearance?

Yes   No   Do you find that you need frequent reassurance about your weight or appearance?

Yes   No   Are you ashamed of your body or your appearance?

Yes   No   Do you wish that you could have cosmetic surgery to correct some flaw in your appearance?

Yes   No   Did your family or friends criticize your weight or appearance when you were a child?

Barriers to Sexuality Phase III

■ BTS 15 (Women)

Around the time of your menstrual period:

Yes   No   Do you experience bloating or weight gain?

Yes   No   Are your breasts tender?

Yes   No   Do you feel anxious or irritable?

Yes   No   Do you cry more easily than usual?

Yes   No   Do you feel excessively tired?

Yes   No   Do you experience food cravings or changes in your appetite?

Yes   No   Do you sleep more or less than you usually do?

Yes   No   Do you have trouble concentrating or remembering things?

Yes   No   Do you experience abdominal pain or changes in your bowel habits?

Yes   No   Do you find that you're less interested in sex than usual?

■ BTS 16 (Women)

Yes   No   Do you have hot flashes?

Yes   No   Do you have breast tenderness?

Yes   No   Have your PMS symptoms worsened?

Yes   No   Do you have decreased libido?

Yes   No   Are your periods irregular?

Yes   No   Do you suffer from fatigue?

Yes   No   Do you have vaginal dryness or discomfort during sex?

Yes   No   Do you have urine leakage when coughing or sneezing?

Yes   No   Do you have mood swings?

Yes   No   Are you having difficulty sleeping?

■ BTS 17 (Women)

Yes	No	Have you ceased menstruating?
Yes	No	Are you suffering from hot flashes?
Yes	No	Do you have mood swings?
Yes	No	Do you have less interest in sex than you used to?
Yes	No	Are you having trouble sleeping?
Yes	No	Do you have a rapid or irregular heartbeat at times?
Yes	No	Are you having joint pain or headaches?

■ BTS 18 (Women)

Yes	No	Are you older than forty-five?
Yes	No	Are you menopausal?
Yes	No	Have you been diagnosed with osteoporosis?
Yes	No	Have you noticed that you're less interested in sex than you once were?
Yes	No	Have you noticed that you rarely think or fantasize about sex?
Yes	No	Do you enjoy sex less than you once did?
Yes	No	Do you have trouble remembering or concentrating more than you once did?
Yes	No	Are you less muscular than you once were?
Yes	No	Do you feel as if your muscles are weaker than they once were?
Yes	No	Have you noticed an increase in your body fat?

■ BTS 19 (Men)

Yes	No	Do you frequently experience fatigue for no apparent reason?
Yes	No	Have your moods been depressed lately?
Yes	No	Have you been more irritable recently?
Yes	No	Are you less focused than you once were?
Yes	No	Do you look less muscular than you once did?
Yes	No	Do you feel as if you're not as strong as you once were?
Yes	No	Do you have more body fat than you once did?
Yes	No	Is your sex drive lower than it once was?
Yes	No	Are you having difficulty achieving or maintaining an erection?
Yes	No	Do you have less facial and body hair than you once did?

Barriers to Sexuality Phase IV (Men and Women)

■ BTS 20

Yes	No	Do you drink alcoholic beverages on a regular basis?
Yes	No	Do you ever find yourself wishing that you could cut down or drink less?
Yes	No	Do you ever find yourself getting angry when someone suggests that you drink less?
Yes	No	Do you ever feel guilty about your drinking?
Yes	No	Do you ever take a drink in the morning as an "eye-opener" or to help you recover from a hangover?

■ BTS 21

Yes	No	Do you find that you're out of breath after climbing a flight of stairs?
Yes	No	Are you frequently tired, even when you haven't engaged in strenuous activity?
Yes	No	Do you find it difficult or impossible to touch your toes?
Yes	No	Do you seldom or rarely exercise?
Yes	No	Do you usually take the elevator instead of the stairs?
Yes	No	Do you feel that you're less energetic than you used to be?
Yes	No	Are you overweight?
Yes	No	Do you feel that you're weaker than you used to be?

■ BTS 22

Yes	No	Do you routinely sleep less than seven hours a night?
Yes	No	Do you feel as if you could easily fall asleep at almost any time during the day?
Yes	No	Do you find yourself nodding off unexpectedly?
Yes	No	Do you feel that you're more irritable lately?
Yes	No	Do you frequently feel tired and run-down during the day?
Yes	No	Do you feel exhausted and ready for bed long before your partner is?
Yes	No	Do you have trouble concentrating?
Yes	No	Are you more forgetful than you once were?
Yes	No	Do you find it difficult to get out of bed in the morning?
Yes	No	Do you feel that you're usually too tired to have sex?

Yes	No	Do you routinely work more than ten hours a day?
Yes	No	Do you find yourself thinking about work when you should be relaxing?
Yes	No	Do you spend your free time on work-related projects?
Yes	No	Do you carry a work-related cell phone or a pager, even when you're "off-duty?"
Yes	No	Has your work ever caused you to miss an important social or family obligation?
Yes	No	Has your work ever caused you to break a promise?
Yes	No	Has your partner ever complained that your job comes before him/her?

■ BTS 24

Yes	No	Do you regularly skip breakfast?
Yes	No	Do you rarely eat three meals a day?
Yes	No	Do you usually eat more than three snacks a day?
Yes	No	Do you frequently skip meals?
Yes	No	Do you find that you are often so hungry that you overeat at mealtime?
Yes	No	Do you eat most of your meals somewhere besides a dining table?
Yes	No	Do you eat more than three meals a week at fast food restaurants?
Yes	No	Do you frequently eat on the go?
Yes	No	Do you frequently graze, or eat continuously?

■ BTS 25

Yes	No	Do you eat fewer than three servings of fruit each day?
Yes	No	Do you eat fewer than three servings of vegetables each day?
Yes	No	Are you on a high-protein diet?
Yes	No	Do you frequently experience food cravings?
Yes	No	Do you often feel sluggish or sleepy after you eat?
Yes	No	Do you often feel hungry soon after eating?
Yes	No	Do you drink fewer than six glasses of water a day?

■ BTS 26

Yes	No	Do you drink more than three cups of regular coffee a day?
Yes	No	Do you drink more than three caffeine-containing soft drinks a day?
Yes	No	Do you find that you're nervous or irritable if you miss your morning coffee?
Yes	No	Do you develop a headache when you miss your morning coffee?
Yes	No	Do you usually drink a cup of coffee or a caffeine-containing soft drink for a "pick me up" during the day?
Yes	No	Do you awaken with a headache on the mornings that you sleep in?

Barriers To Sexuality Phase V (Men and Women)

■ BTS 27

Yes	No	Do you have less interest in sex than you once did?
Yes	No	Do you find that you rarely or never think or fantasize about sex?
Yes	No	Do you find that you rarely or never initiate sex with your partner?
Yes	No	Do you have sex just to please your partner?
Yes	No	Has your partner expressed concern about your lack of sexual desire?
Yes	No	Is your lack of sexual desire causing problems in your relationship?
Yes	No	Do you wish that you were more interested in sex?
Yes	No	Have you ever experienced a traumatic sexual encounter?
Yes	No	Were you taught as a child that sex is shameful or sinful?

■ BTS 28

Yes	No	Do you have little interest in sex?
Yes	No	Do you rarely or never experience orgasm with sexual intercourse?
Yes	No	Are you rarely or never able to achieve orgasm by any means?
Yes	No	Do you take an antidepressant or sedative medication?
Yes	No	Do you have a history of drug or alcohol abuse?

■ BTS 29 (Women)

Yes	No	Do you suffer from depression or anxiety?
Yes	No	Do you have a chronic illness, like heart disease, lung disease, or diabetes?
Yes	No	Do you have a history of drug or alcohol abuse?
Yes	No	Do you take antidepressant medications?
Yes	No	Are you having marital or relationship problems?
Yes	No	Do you have a history of sexual abuse?
Yes	No	Are you unable to experience orgasm?
Yes	No	Do you experience pain during sexual intercourse?
Yes	No	Do you have little interest in having sex?
Yes	No	Do you feel that you have inadequate vaginal lubrication?

■ BTS 30 (Women)

Yes	No	Do you have pelvic pain with intercourse, especially when your partner thrusts?
Yes	No	Are you menopausal?
Yes	No	Do you suffer from frequent vaginal infections?
Yes	No	Have you had a C-section?
Yes	No	Have you had a hysterectomy?
Yes	No	Have you had a bilateral tubal ligation (tubes tied)?
Yes	No	Have you had abdominal surgery?
Yes	No	Have you ever been diagnosed with pelvic inflammatory disease?
Yes	No	Has it been more than two years since you had a pelvic exam?
Yes	No	Do you suffer from vaginal dryness?

■ BTS 31 (Women)

Yes	No	Do you experience vaginal pain with penetration?Do you feel that penetration is difficult or impossible at times?
Yes	No	Do you fear that sexual intercourse will be painful?
Yes	No	Do you have a history of sexual trauma, including rape or sexual abuse as a child?
Yes	No	Have you ever experienced feelings of panic or extreme anxiety prior to or during sexual intercourse?

■ BTS 32 (Men)

Yes	No	Are you younger than thirty?
Yes	No	Do you frequently ejaculate before you want to?
Yes	No	Do you usually experience orgasm before your partner does?
Yes	No	Do you feel that you are unable to stop yourself from climaxing, even for a few seconds?
Yes	No	Were you taught as a child that sex is shameful or sinful?
Yes	No	Do you frequently experience feelings of guilt about having sex?

■ BTS 33 (Men)

Yes	No	Do you sometimes fail to get an erection during sexual activity?
Yes	No	Do you sometimes fail to maintain an erection during sexual activity?
Yes	No	Do you feel that your erection is less firm than it once was?
Yes	No	Do you feel that you are having problems or turmoil in your relationship?
Yes	No	Do you smoke?
Yes	No	Are you older than fifty?
Yes	No	Do you have diabetes?
Yes	No	Do you have high blood pressure?
Yes	No	Do you have high cholesterol?
Yes	No	Do you take medication for depression, high cholesterol, or high blood pressure?

Barriers to Sexuality Phase VI

■ BTS 34 (Men)

Yes	No	I have a hard time making small talk with my partner.
Yes	No	When my partner tells me about her problems, I find myself offering her solutions instead of encouraging her to discuss them.
Yes	No	I tend to "show" my partner my love, rather than "tell" her.
Yes	No	I have trouble discussing my feelings with my partner.
Yes	No	I feel that making love is a reasonable substitute for conversation.

■ BTS 35 (Women)

Yes	No	I try to engage my partner in small talk, even when he's not in the mood for conversation.
Yes	No	I try to get my partner to "open up" and discuss his problems or concerns, even if it makes him uncomfortable.
Yes	No	I tend to tell my partner that I love him more often than I show him.
Yes	No	I think conversation is a reasonable substitute for making love.

Barriers to Sexuality Phase VII (Men and Women)

To answer the questions for BTS 36 through BTS 45, circle the number that reflects the following statements:

1—Strongly agree
2—Somewhat agree
3—Neither agree nor disagree
4—Somewhat disagree
5—Strongly disagree

■ BTS 36

1	2	3	4	5	My usual sexual encounter is a "quickie."
1	2	3	4	5	I find it difficult to make time in my schedule to make love to my partner.
1	2	3	4	5	Sex is last on my "to do" list.
1	2	3	4	5	I rarely think about making love to my partner.
1	2	3	4	5	I hardly ever initiate sexual activity.

■ BTS 37

1	2	3	4	5	I do not think of myself as being a sexual person.
1	2	3	4	5	I seldom wear clothes that make me feel sexy.
1	2	3	4	5	I do not flirt with my partner.
1	2	3	4	5	I rarely have sexual thoughts or fantasies.
1	2	3	4	5	I'm not sure what it takes to make me feel sexy.

■ BTS 38

1	2	3	4	5	Having sex feels like a chore.
1	2	3	4	5	When my partner and I make love, I know just what to expect.
1	2	3	4	5	My partner and I make love in the same location.
1	2	3	4	5	My partner and I rarely try new sexual positions.
1	2	3	4	5	I find it difficult to get excited about having sex with my partner.

■ BTS 39

1	2	3	4	5	My partner and I rarely spend time alone with each other.
1	2	3	4	5	When my partner and I are together, we usually talk about our jobs, our children, or our finances.
1	2	3	4	5	My partner and I rarely make eye contact with each other.
1	2	3	4	5	My partner and I seldom laugh together.
1	2	3	4	5	I can't remember the last time my partner and I went out on a "date."

■ BTS 40

1	2	3	4	5	My partner and I disagree about the "right" amount of sexual activity.
1	2	3	4	5	My partner and I frequently have arguments about sex.
1	2	3	4	5	When we have sex, one of us is usually motivated by feelings of guilt.
1	2	3	4	5	When we have sex, one of usually ends up feeling resentful or "used."
1	2	3	4	5	In our relationship, the same partner usually initiates lovemaking.

Barriers to Sexuality
Phase VIII (Men and Women)

■ **BTS 41**

1 2 3 4 5   In terms of our relationship, I feel that my partner and I are not equally committed.

1 2 3 4 5   One of us contributes more to our relationship than the other.

1 2 3 4 5   My partner fails to keep his/her promises to me.

1 2 3 4 5   I do not think that my partner and I will be together in five years.

1 2 3 4 5   When we are angry with each other, my partner and I discuss ending our relationship.

■ **BTS 42**

1 2 3 4 5   I feel that my partner does not value my contributions to our relationship.

1 2 3 4 5   I feel that my partner is taking advantage of me.

1 2 3 4 5   I feel that my partner does not value my feelings or opinions.

1 2 3 4 5   My partner does not respect my time and my obligations outside of our relationship.

1 2 3 4 5   My partner does not treat me with respect around other people.

■ BTS 43

1 2 3 4 5	My partner does not notice when he/she has hurt my feelings.
1 2 3 4 5	My partner gives me the "silent treatment" to punish me or to get even with me.
1 2 3 4 5	I feel that my partner expects me to read his/her mind.
1 2 3 4 5	I feel like I never know what is going on in my partner's life.
1 2 3 4 5	I feel that my partner doesn't listen to my concerns, ideas, and problems with genuine interest.

■ BTS 44

1 2 3 4 5	I feel that I cannot freely express my feelings to my partner.
1 2 3 4 5	I am afraid to be totally honest with my partner.
1 2 3 4 5	I feel that my partner might consider having an affair.
1 2 3 4 5	My partner isn't always honest with me.
1 2 3 4 5	I feel that my partner keeps secrets from me.

■ BTS 45

1 2 3 4 5	My partner and I usually sit apart from each other when we're at home together.
1 2 3 4 5	My partner and I do not hug each other every day.
1 2 3 4 5	My partner and I rarely hold hands when we're walking together.
1 2 3 4 5	My partner and I sleep in separate beds.
1 2 3 4 5	My partner and I seldom touch each other playfully or lovingly.

BTS Phase I:
Diseases and Disorders in Men and Women

The questions for BTS 1 through BTS 11 pertain to risk factors for the following diseases or disorders. While even a single "yes" answer to any one of the listed questions can increase your likelihood of having or developing the relevant disease or disorder, the more questions you answer in the affirmative, the greater your chances of having or developing the relevant disease or disorder. Be sure to discuss your findings and your concerns with your physician.

Each of these conditions has the potential to lower your sex drive. In Chapters 4-8, I explain how, and tell you the steps you can take to eliminate—or at least minimize—the impact.

BTS 1: Heart disease (See page 87.)

BTS 2: Diabetes (See page 89.)

BTS 3: High cholesterol (See page 91.)

BTS 4: Hypertension (high blood pressure) (See page 93.)

BTS 5: Hypothyroidism (low thyroid hormone) (See page 98.)

BTS 6: Hyperthyroidism (elevated thyroid hormone) (See page 98.)

BTS 7: Chronic fatigue syndrome (See page 99.)

BTS 8: Obstructive sleep apnea (See page 130.)

BTS 9: Medication side effects (See page 139.)

BTS 10: Urinary incontinence in women (See page 121.)

BTS 11: Benign prostatic hyperplasia (BPH) in men (See page 125.)

BTS Phase II:
Emotional Disorders in Men and Women

The questions for BTS 12 through BTS 14 will help you identify emotional disorders that may be interfering with your libido or sexual performance. The more positive responses you have, the greater the likelihood that you're suffering from an emotional disorder. If you feel that you are at risk for the following conditions, it is important to discuss your concerns with your doctor or a mental health professional.

BTS 12: Depression (See page 102.)

BTS 13: Chronic stress (See page 171.)

BTS 14: Poor body image (See page 190.)

BTS Phase III:
Hormonal Imbalance

Affirmative responses to the questions for BTS 15 through BTS 19 may point to a hormonal imbalance, but the final diagnosis will likely depend on the results of blood tests and a physical examination.

Women

BTS 15: Premenstrual syndrome (PMS) or Premenstrual dysphoric disorder (PMDD) (See page 105-109.)

BTS 16: Perimenopause (See page 112.)

BTS 17: Menopause (See page 115.)

BTS 18: Testosterone deficiency (See page 117.)

Men

BTS 19: Andropause (See page 135.)

BTS Phase IV: Lifestyle Issues

If you answered "yes" to any of the questions for BTS 19 through BTS 25, lifestyle issues could be at the root of your diminished desire or suboptimal sexual performance. While you should definitely involve your doctor in addressing alcohol dependency, you can usually conquer the other lifestyle issues on your own.

BTS 20: Alcohol dependency (See page 177.)

BTS 21: Poor physical conditioning (See page 193.)

BTS 22: Sleep deprivation (See page 167.)

BTS 23: Overwork syndrome (See page 12.)

BTS 24: Poor eating habits (See page 201.)

BTS 25: Poor nutritional balance (See page 201.)

BTS 26: Caffeine dependency (See page 179.)

BTS Phase V: Sexual Dysfunction

The questions for BTS 27 through 33 are designed to help you determine if a sexual dysfunction is at the root of diminished desire or performance problems. If you answered "yes" to one or more of the questions in this section, and you suspect that you have one of the following conditions, your physician will be able to confirm the diagnosis and recommend the appropriate treatments.

BTS 27: Hypoactive sexual desire disorder (HSDD) (See page 68.)

BTS 28: Orgasmic disorder (See page 82.)

Women

BTS 29: Female sexual arousal disorder (FSAD) (See page 79.)

BTS 30: Dyspareunia (See page 76.)

BTS 31: Vaginismus (See page 78.)

Men

BTS 32: Premature ejaculation (See page 75.)

BTS 33: Erectile dysfunction (See page 71.)

Phase VI: Conversation Style

BTS 34: Right-brain conversationalist (See page 58.)

BTS 35: Left-brain conversationalist (See page 58.)

Phase VII: Sexuality Issues

BTS 36 through 40 will help you uncover sexuality issues that may needsome work. Add your scores for each BTS, and then use the following grading system:

Score	Evaluation
1-15	Needs immediate attention
9-16	Needs improvement
17-25	Not a problem

BTS 36: Sexuality is not a priority

BTS 37: Sexual identity issues

BTS 38: Your sex life is in a rut

BTS 39: Intimacy deficit

BTS 40: Desire discrepancy (See Chapter 3.)

Phase VIII: Relationship Issues

BTS 41 through 45 will help you identify barriers to sexuality in your relationship. Use the same grading scale as above.

BTS 41: Commitment

BTS 42: Respect

BTS 43: Communication

BTS 44: Trust

BTS 45: Touch